P9-BBP-927

# Men Are Stupid . . .
# And They Like Big Boobs

A Woman's Guide to Beauty Through Plastic Surgery

# Men Are Stupid . . .
# And They Like Big Boobs

A Woman's Guide to Beauty Through Plastic Surgery

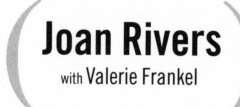

# Joan Rivers

with Valerie Frankel

**Pocket Books**

New York   London   Toronto   Sydney

Pocket Books
A Division of Simon & Schuster, Inc.
1230 Avenue of the Americas
New York, NY 10020

Regarding plastic surgery and non-invasive cosmetic procedures, each patient's needs
and requirements are unique. Each doctor has his and her particular methods and
strategies. Therefore, we have described surgeries and procedures in general "standard"
terms. For specific details about surgeries and procedures as they apply to an individual
patient or client, consult a doctor. Consult two or three. Read this book with the under-
standing that your surgery might not proceed *exactly* as we've described it here.

First Pocket Books hardcover edition January 2009

POCKET and colophon are registered trademarks of Simon & Schuster, Inc.

For information about special discounts for bulk purchases,
please contact Simon & Schuster Special Sales at 1-800-456-6798
or business@simonandschuster.com

Designed by Ruth Lee Mui

Manufactured in the United States of America

10   9   8   7   6   5   4   3   2   1

Library of Congress Cataloging-in-Publication Data is available.

ISBN-13: 978-1-4165-9922-7
ISBN-10:     1-4165-9922-3

This book is dedicated to all the women who've felt they had to keep their plastic surgery a secret, who've lied about having had it, and who've felt shame about needing it, wanting it, or doing it. May you never have a moment's guilt and embarrassment again, only pride in your appearance and joy about how you feel.

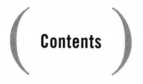

# ( Contents )

*Asterisks indicate chapters that include procedures I've done personally.†
†That's a lot of asterisks!

# Men Are Stupid . . .
# And They Like Big Boobs

A Woman's Guide to Beauty Through Plastic Surgery

# **Welcome** to My World

Okay, politically incorrect or not, let's face it, men are stupid. They can't help it. They're wired to procreate and Mother Nature has doomed the poor things. They are attracted to creatures that are their opposites, with hairless bodies, big boobs, slim waists, rounded butts—and this has become the beauty ideal many women aspire to achieve.

So why not? Aren't we past the age of "I can do everything; I don't need a man?" Nowadays, it's "I can do everything, *and* I want a man— *and* I want to be beautiful." Or, it's "Yes, I'm smart. Yes, I'm educated. And *yes*, I still want to feel the thrill of looking in the mirror and liking what I see."

When people used to say a woman was smart, it was a nice way of saying she was ugly. Beautiful women were often assumed to be stupid. These days, smart means just that—smart. And beautiful means just that—beautiful. No one cares how a woman got that way, just as long as she is. I think women shouldn't settle for less than being both smart *and* beautiful. For many of us, having it all means getting a nip, or a tuck, or a little lift now and again. Why? Because it makes us feel good.

I was talking with a rich friend last year and said that I wanted to write a book about beauty and cosmetic surgery. It would be part personal history, part insight, and part practical advice about treatments. My rich friend said, "Great idea. Get to work. Can't wait to read it. And send me a freebie."*

I've been the public (lifted) face of cosmetic enhancement since the Stone Age. My luck was to realize early on the degree to which looking good helped my life and career—and to start having work done early, too. My abiding life philosophy is plain: *In our appearance-centric society, beauty is a huge factor in everyone's professional and emotional success*—for good or ill, it's the way things are; accept it or go live under a rock.

In our society, looks matter more than anyone would like to believe, and it's senseless to go through life angry about it when you can just embrace it. Looking good equals *feeling* good. Feeling good equals having more confidence. So why not do whatever you can to improve your appearance? Unlike a dress that goes out of style, or a diet that ultimately fails, a beautiful nose is forever. You can get mad about society's demands, you can say, "I'm proud of the way God made me," or you can get beautiful.

Some people feel I have had too much plastic surgery, whereas others feel I could probably still use some more work. Most just don't care. I tend to agree with the latter group, then again, screw'em all. I feel like Joan Rivers.

The title of this book, *Men Are Stupid . . . And They Like Big Boobs,*

---

*That's why my friend is rich.

is something that was said to me by Marilyn Monroe herself,* and she was right! It was as true then as it is now.

Let's face it. Men are guided not by their brains, but by their eyes and penises. A man looks at an attractive woman and thinks, "I'd tap that." A woman looks at herself and thinks about her flaws and the guilt she feels about hating them. She might try to rally her spirits around her inner beauty. We've been taught since kindergarten that the quest for inner beauty is noble and powerful, while pursuing outer beauty is vain and superficial and not nearly as empowering as achieving a really good personality. Yet, come on! Despite a woman's bedrock belief in her inner goodness, her eyes keep drifting back to her wrinkles, or her big nose, or her belly roll. The truth is, inner beauty might get you a promotion, or, for that matter, a raise, but it won't get you a husband, or a lover. No one ever asked Eleanor Roosevelt to dance. Except maybe Gertrude Stein.

Relax. You shouldn't have mixed emotions about wanting to be sexy and gorgeous. It's normal! No one gets up in the morning and says, "Hey, what can I do today to turn myself into a dog?" Even the Elephant Man's sister put on lipstick. You're not a selfish, amoral person if you spend money on your appearance. I truly believe that within her means, every woman should do whatever she can to look her best. And she should enjoy doing it, too! Beauty is important, noble, and a requirement for success in our society. Contrary to conventional wisdom, even smart girls are allowed to have—and flaunt—round, perky butts. And a high, hard rear end is a thing of beauty—and a thing we can all have.

In the old days, before cosmetic surgery, the secret of staying young was simply to die early. Nowadays, it's available to anyone with some money and a good doctor.

On these pages, you will enter a golden, modern world full of

---

*Actually, what she said was, "Young woman, men are like moonshiners. Their lives would be meaningless without jugs. Now stop stalking me or I'll call the cops."

miraculous sights and sounds to amaze you—the world of surgical and non-invasive cosmetic procedures.

Or, what I call The Home Planet.

Most women are curious about it. Who hasn't fantasized about having Botox Cosmetic injections or a face lift or a boob job? Of the nation's 150 million women, I'll bet 149,999,999* of them have dreamed of making some kind of beauty change. What I've done is present to you just about every procedure that's being legally performed in America today, explained in language that I—and therefore, you—can understand, even after a two-martini lunch. And I won't hold back. (Have I ever?) The explanation of how an implant goes from a cold steel table to a bra cup will make you salivate.

I'm not saying cosmetic intervention is right for everyone. I've always believed that, for some women the best beauty aid in the world is getting married; for others, it's getting divorced. For me? The best beauty aid would be getting blackmail-quality photographs of a plastic surgeon.

## A Very, Very Brief History of Plastic Surgery

The ancient Egyptians were the first civilization to do just about *anything*, and that included skin grafts to repair facial damage and crude nose jobs (inspired by the Sphinx, perhaps?), circa 4000 B.C.

The earliest example of an official doctor's "chart" was written—probably, illegibly—in Sanskrit by the Indian surgeon Sushruta in 600 B.C., who recorded his experiments with the above-mentioned nose jobs, skin grafts, and other facial reconstructions. All performed without anesthesia. Those women were dedicated!

The Greeks and Romans improved on these techniques. In the first century B.C., Aulus Cornelius Celsus wrote volumes about re-

*And that's not including cross-dressers and post-op trannies.

constructing ears, lips, and noses that would hold up, in terms of anatomical accuracy, today.

In 350 A.D., the first multi-volume encyclopedia of medicine was composed by Oribasius, the personal physician of the Roman emperor Julian the Apostate. He included details about all the known history of reconstructive surgery: facial deformities, cartilage, and detailed anatomy of the nose and ears.

Then the story of plastic surgery stalls for about a thousand years during the Dark Ages. The spread of Christianity, alas, was to blame. Back then, tampering with the body was considered a sin against God, and surgery was thought of as the devil's work. Thank God, the groundbreaking work of the ancients wasn't forgotten by surgeons who—for the benefit of women like me—practiced in secret and passed their knowledge from generation to generation, even though they risked their lives to do so.

Then, in the year 1200, Pope Innocent III prohibited all surgery, which, unfortunately, ushered in the tradition of homely nuns.

The Renaissance kick-started the study of anatomy and medicine again around the world. In 1465, a Turk named Sharafeddin Sabuncuoglu published the *Imperial Surgery*, which described rudimentary oral surgery, eyelid lifts, and breast reduction. Around the same time, in Germany, Heinrich von Pfolspeundt wrote about nose reconstruction. In Italy, several fifteenth-century surgeons performed rhinoplasties, risking excommunication from the Church.

But plastic surgery didn't become more common, however, for another few hundred years. The main reason? Pain. Worse than the kind you get from seeing yourself naked.

Before the nineteenth century, surgeries were done without any anesthesia. Once doctors started using carbon dioxide, nitrous oxide, and ether in the early 1800s, plastic surgery techniques improved greatly, mainly in Western Europe. Nose jobs, skin grafts, bone grafts, and lip and ear reconstructions were being done all over the continent, and, by mid-century, in America. The first American plastic surgeon was named John Peter Mettaur, and he made history by doing the first ever cleft palate operation in 1829. Eugene Hollander did the first face lift in Berlin in 1901.

As is often the case, necessity spurred innovation. The biggest advances in the field were the consequence of war and improvements in modern weaponry. Surgeons had to invent ways to repair never-seen-before injuries to the faces and bodies of soldiers. Improvements continued to move at a breakneck pace for decades, notably burn treatments on soldiers during World War II.

Until the late twentieth century, the emphasis of plastic surgery was reconstruction. The shift toward cosmetic surgery came about in the 1960s, when early breast implants were developed—saline implants in France, silicone gel implants in America. Liposuction was invented around this time in Europe. Tummy tucks, body lifts, refinements, and advances in every possible cosmetic technique moved along at a breakneck pace during the 1970s, and continue to evolve, at increasing speed, today.

Thank God!

The women of tomorrow will never again be subjected to taunting, name-calling, or public ostracizing, unless, of course, they choose to be seen with Russell Crowe.

## My Own History with Plastic Surgery (Have You Got a Couple of Hours?)

I've been asked many times to list all the procedures I've done, spread out over forty years. To the best of my recollection, here's the rundown:

When I was in college, I had my first procedure. My nose was chubby, and I had it thinned. I went with my mother to see the doctor in Manhattan, got a local anesthetic, and had my nose thinned (I remember the sound of the file, or whatever they used). They put an ice pack on my face, and then I took the train home afterward with my mother. It was so easy, so relatively painless that it left me with a great impression, not to mention a thinner nose.

When I was in my late thirties, I had my eyes done. Just like my father, I had big bags under my eyes that really bothered me. Melissa, my daughter, was a baby. I was doing the Johnny Carson show, and seeing the bags on TV really horrified me. I'll never forget, a French singer—a cute little cupcake named Geneviève who appeared on the show—said to me, "Do your eyes now, when you're young, so no one will know." I went and had the bags removed with the eye lift. And she was right. No one knew. People just said about me, "Success makes her look better."

I remember I took Melissa to Fire Island right after the surgery. I had terrible black eyes. Someone asked, "What happened?" I said, "My baby punched me!"

A few years later, I appeared for the first time on the cover of *People* magazine. I didn't like how my nose looked. It was droopy, so I went and had it done again, this time not to make it thinner, but to slightly raise the tip. The doctor who did the surgery had the issue of *People* in his waiting room. He said, laughing, "I have to make you look like you, but not you." And that's exactly what he did. He got rid of the droop, and I still looked like the cover photo, only better.

Now *that's* good plastic surgery!

I had my first full face lift when I was in my early forties. It was 1975. In those days, face lifts were a) not talked about, and b) done in a hospital. Patients would spend two days there post-op before they let them go home. I came out of the operating room wrapped up like a mummy around my head, my eyes bruised, lips swollen, feeling very groggy, but by my second day, I was up and about. While taking a stroll down the hospital corridor, I saw two women I knew dressed in gorgeous silk robes also walking around the floor, bandaged exactly like I was. I greeted them happily and asked what they had done. Face? Eyes? What? Both insisted they'd been in separate car accidents! I guess we were *all* in car accidents. And we all got banged up in *exactly* the same places on the face.

In the early 1980s, liposuction was getting popular in America. It was very exciting, this great new procedure to get rid of fat in an hour. A friend of mine got lipo on her chin to sharpen her jawline, and she looked beautiful afterward.

I had bigger saddlebags than the Pony Express (those bulges on my thighs made me look like I was wearing permanent jodhpurs), so I decided to have them lipo'ed.

The fat was vacuumed out, and my thighs looked great. But later I got new bumps of fat around my waist. Lipo technique has since improved, as has nearly every procedure I've tried—*after* I did it, of course.

I had a breast reduction operation next. Odd, you might think, when you consider my act at the time. I said I started out with tiny boobs, and I had big jokes about them, such as "I'd go to the beach, and people would think I was selling Milk Duds" or "On my honeymoon, I came naked into the room, and my husband said, 'Can I help you with the buttons?' " But then after I had Melissa, my boobs started growing, and growing, and growing, and I woke up one day with major bazonkas.

With breasts, it all comes down to schtupping and fashion. When I cared more about schtupping and wanted big breasts, I didn't have them. When I cared about fashion and didn't want them, I got massive big boobs. I would try on amazing, expensive dresses, and my boobs would muffin-top all over the place.

I signed up for a breast reduction. I went down two cup sizes, and I loved it.

The next big operation I had was a tummy tuck. This happened by accident! I swear! I was scheduled for a hysterectomy, and I told the gynecological surgeon I wanted a plastic surgeon to come in after and finish the job. At the time, this was totally unheard of. It might have offended the ob/gyn surgeon's ego to suggest I wouldn't like his stitching.

By the way, *never* worry about offending a doctor's ego. He'll go home after the surgery and play golf, pretending your head is the golf ball. But you're stuck with a bad scar for the rest of your life.

Always, if possible, have a plastic surgeon do your stitching. I was the only hysterectomy patient smiling in the recovery room that day. The others were all sobbing about never being able to have another baby, while I was loving the look of my flat new belly, laughing and saying, "Where's my bikini?"

From that point on, my plastic surgery journey became a series of minor tweaks here and there: maintenance stuff, like polishing the car or keeping the house painted. The muscles under my chin got loose from talking, and I needed a clean jawline. A wobbly under-chin is a giveaway of a woman's age. I've had it cleaned up three times, the last being three years ago. My lower eyelids never got puffy after my first eye lift all those years ago, but I did have my upper eyelids done after my first face lift.

Every six months or so, I go in for my Botox Cosmetic* shots, collagen in my lips, and if I have something to burn off, a mark or spot, I do it. I've also had a chemical peel that a dear friend gave me as a surprise. It was the only procedure that has ever been painful. Last year, I had my upper arms lipo'ed so they'd look skinny in sweaters.

If anything else comes up that sounds great, I'll probably try it. Why not? Looking good is not the sin of vanity. Looking good is the virtue of diligence! Many think of surgery as morally wrong or messing with a divine plan.

A lot of women have come up to me and said, "God created this nose." To which I respond, "And he also created plastic surgeons to fix it."

---

*Botox Cosmetic, not Botox. I'll explain later.

## Surgery Is Out of the Closet—Sort Of

Weirdly, people will tell you the most intimate things about their sex lives and money, but clam up about plastic surgery. It truly annoys me when celebrities, models, and movie stars take advantage of what's available, and then deny having done it, as if it's their great shame to have been born with flaws. As if only "natural" beauty is valid.

It's truly insane that the very same celebrities who sob at interview after interview about going into rehab or their stay in jail still refuse to talk about tweaking their noses or raising their brows.

Comediennes—women like Roseanne Barr, Phyllis Diller, Kathy Griffin, Carol Burnett, and me, who aren't required to be beautiful but still want to look good—we're the ones who have come out. A few other celebrities have been waving the banner along with them. Cher is very outspoken on the subject, even joking that she's had so much done and added to her face that when she dies, she'll be donating her body to Tupperware.

Dolly Parton has always been truthful about her multiple procedures. She's had *everything* lifted. If she wants to give you the finger, she has to flip you the toe.

Pamela Anderson—good for her!—has never pretended like those were her real boobs, making them bigger, then smaller, then bigger. She's gone under the knife more times than a Butterball turkey.

Demi Moore spent an alleged $500,000 getting head-to-toe plastic surgery—and she earned a handsome younger husband out of that investment! More and more public figures are coming out about their surgeries, especially the new generation of stars: Ashlee Simpson (nose), Beyoncé (nose), Paris Hilton (lips). Tyra Banks shares my belief that surgery levels the playing field. Why shouldn't *everyone* be beautiful? That democratic notion has come of age.

And how lucky are we to be living in an age when cosmetic surgery has finally gone mainstream? Botox Cosmetic injections are as accepted as manicures; nose jobs are as commonplace as braces.

Nearly twelve million cosmetic surgical and minimally invasive pro-cedures were performed in 2007, a nearly 500 percent increase since 1997. Doctors and forecasters agree that the numbers will continue to rise. And wouldn't it be wonderful if, like in Brazil where plastic surgery is free, instead of keeping their treatment a secret, women will brag about what they had done? Happy women make happy homes and families. They're better neighbors, colleagues, bosses, and friends. Joy and confidence spread like wildfire.

Is there a downside to the mainstreaming of cosmetic surgery? Only perhaps that where there was once too little information about it, now there's too much. There are a dozen "makeover" TV reality shows about plastic surgeons. On any given evening, you can watch celebrities and real people having tummy tucks and face lifts in your living room. There are literally dozens of fillers and lasers, and it's hard to sort out what's right for you. The abundance of information can be overwhelming, which is the reason I wrote this book: to ex-plain to women what's out there and help them figure out their op-tions.

Any woman, of any age, who wants to feel better, look better for her age—not necessarily younger—and has the desire to take steps, will find answers on these pages. My aim is to connect with honest women who feel bad about their necks, as well as their tummies, breasts, acne scars, noses, eyelids, crow's feet, and bubble butts. So many women—and men, too—are desperate for non-intimidating, accessible information on plastic surgery, and I'm just the woman to give it to them. Along with my experience under the knife, I've talked and talked to others who have done the same things I have. I've ac-cumulated a truckload of wisdom about plastic surgery, as a life phi-losophy and on practical terms—and I'm ready to share.

One last thing: I've organized this book to start out small, easy does it, with the toe-in-the-water procedures like wrinkle-filler in-jections, laser hair removal, and skin-resurfacing peels. Then I wade in deeper, with more complicated procedures like face lifts, boob jobs, nose jobs, liposuction. By the time I get to tummy tucks and vagina lifts, you'll be able to talk to a plastic surgeon like you've had eight years of medical school yourself. You can read this book cover to cover, or go directly to the procedure you're particularly curious about, or you can start at the end and work your way to the front. You can start in the middle and skip around. It's your book! You can read it any way you like! You can use it as a doorstop if you want. You can frame the cover and hang it on the wall. It's up to you. That's my ultimate point! Do whatever you want, if it makes you happy.

But first! Take this quiz.

## ( Quiz )

### So You Think You're Really, *Really* Ready for Cosmetic Surgery?

Answer the following multiple-choice questions to find out if you're emotionally prepared to make a big change.

1. **Spending money on myself . . .**
   a. is morally reprehensible!
   b. runs against everything my parents taught me.
   c. is fine. What else should I spend it on? My kids' college education?
   d. is a tough call, but being happy is worth any price.

If you answered a., that spending money on yourself is morally wrong, then get back inside the convent, and pray for me because I'm clearly bound for hell. Even Mel Gibson pays for his own SS uniforms. If you answered c., remind yourself that spending money is good.

The correct answer is d., that there's no better investment than your own confidence and happiness.

2. **I want to make a change in my appearance because . . .**
   a. my husband has been begging me to get implants since his secretary died.
   b. my friend told me every attractive woman has had something done.
   c. I've hated my nose for years, and I'm sick of walking into parties backwards.
   d. when I saw myself in a recent photo, I looked like my mother.

If you answered a. or b., you're wrong. Screw your boob-loving husband and peer-pressuring friend. The one and only reason to get surgery or a non-invasive beauty procedure is for *yourself*. If you think having work done will make you a happier, more confident, contented person, go for it.

If you answered d., you're still wrong. Those of you who have the fear that you're turning into your mother, make a shrink appointment. In the meantime, guess what? Surgery won't alter your genetic code. Even if you've had a face lift, you'll probably *still* look like your mother. (This drives my daughter Melissa crazy.)

The correct response is c., because the motivation for change has to come from inside you.

3. **The actual surgery will be . . .**
   a. a snap.
   b. the first day of a completely different life.
   c. rough. It's major surgery and should be taken seriously.
   d. a bloody nightmare. I don't know how I let Joan Rivers talk me into this.

The correct answer is c. Plastic surgery, from a brow lift to a butt lift, is major surgery and not to be taken lightly. You have to be prepared to do whatever your doctor instructs you to do, before surgery and during the recovery. You're looking at up to a month of convalescence. It's not a walk in the park. But, once the recovery is over, you'll be thrilled you had the surgery.

The one thing you hear most from women who've had cosmetic intervention: "I wish I'd done it sooner."

### 4. Self-improvement is . . .

a. selfish vanity.

b. what we should all strive for throughout our lives, physically, emotionally, mentally. Otherwise, why not just crawl under a rock?

c. impossible. I'm already as good as I'm ever going to get.

d. embarrassing. I'm loathe to reveal my insecurities and flaws to myself, let alone a stranger, especially an attractive doctor.

The correct answer is b. Of course we should strive to improve ourselves! The pursuit of betterment is hardly selfish vanity! Do we educate ourselves out of vanity? Do we expose ourselves to culture to be selfish? Physical improvement via cosmetic intervention is on a par with going to the gym, which most people consider to be masochistic but not vain. Vanity is thinking you're already perfect. And if you're perfect, put this book down and leave the rest of us humans alone.

### 5. Beauty is . . .

a. an unfair societal demand put on women so makeup companies, plastic surgeons, diet-pill manufacturers, and hair salons can stay in business and make tons of money.

b. in the eye of the beholder. When I see a beautiful woman walking down the street, I'm so jealous I want to spit—in her eye.

c. for the very young and/or the very rich.

d. within your grasp, a worthy goal, the way to feel good about yourself and stay vital in the world.

Beauty can be a source of a.) anger, b.) jealousy, and c.) envy. You wouldn't have those negative emotions if you felt beautiful yourself. Imagine being free of jealousy, envy, and anger—and not having first woken up dead and found yourself an angel.

Those who answered d. understand that beauty is within your grasp. Now go out there and get some!

( **One** )

# Hello, Doctor!

Once upon a time, there was an average-looking girl named Joan living with her mother in Brooklyn. Joan did not have a boyfriend or much of a social life—lately she'd been sitting home collecting more dust than a Swiffer. Concerned, her mother took Joan to see the Broadway show Grey Gardens, a lighthearted little musical about a mother and a daughter who, in their youth, had bright futures but wound up spinsters living together in a dilapidated old mansion and pretending cat food was pâté. Horrified, Joan and her mother, "Big Joan," left the show fearful of their own futures.

The next night, still worried that her daughter might wind up dancing on the front porch wearing a turban made out of a t-shirt fastened to her head with a diamond brooch, Joan's mother settled in to watch "Extreme Makeover–Home Edition." Hours later, after the makeover's reveal and getting a tad bit tipsy on a second glass of vino, she came to an amazing epiphany: what her daughter needed was a makeover! An Extreme Make-over from the ground up! She knew her sweet, kind daughter might have a *great foundation, but it was time to rip all the boards off the structure and start from scratch.*

*Helpfully and generously, Joan's mother suggested a head-to-toe makeover and cosmetic surgery to her loving daughter. She reached into her bra and removed wads of cash to give to her.*

*Joan was thrilled about the money her mother presented for her makeover, but she decided in a flash that she wasn't going to waste her inheritance on cosmetic surgery.*

*Even though Joan wanted to take her mother's advice, in actuality she was terrified at the thought of going under the knife. She hated knives! She had always believed knives were dangerous, which is why she had never eaten at Benihana or paid to see a Las Vegas magic act. So, Joan insisted on bypassing all professional beauty facilitators and doing the makeover herself. She was good at fixer-uppers and scrapbooking and crafting, so this should be a piece of cake, she thought. But this is where her problems began.*

Quick: Name one thing that you want done really well but can't do by yourself.

Besides sex, it's cosmetic surgery. And in order to have the best result, you need a great doctor.

The most important partner you'll choose in your entire life is, hand to God, your plastic surgeon—the man or woman who holds your life and looks in his or her hands, literally. (Henceforth, I'll be using "his" and "he" for convenience, and not because I think men are better at poking, slicing, and peeling, as I don't. We all know women have excellent knife skills—ask Lorena Bobbitt.)

Why do you need to have enormous trust and faith in your doctor or dermatologist (or, as I like to call him, your beauty facilitator)? Easy. If you buy a dress and then decide it's hideous, you can return it. But if you get bum Botox Cosmetic injections, you're stuck with the Kabuki mask-like face for months. A bad hair cut is temporary; a nose job could be forever. Your choice in doctor or dermatologist is perhaps the only time in your life when you *must* get it right the first time.

The trick is learning how to sift through the dross to find the good guys. It's tough sledding; I know. There are so many doctors doing plastic surgery in Los Angeles that if you haven't been approached by one, you *are* one. The California flag has stars and sutures, for God's sake.

And New York City is just as bad. People used to shoot up heroin in alleyways. Nowadays, they shoot up Botox Cosmetic in living rooms.

You've heard plenty regarding plastic surgery train wrecks like Tara Reid and Courtney Love, about how people with all the money in the world make such bad choices when it comes to picking their doctors? The reason is simple: *They don't do their homework.* You, darling reader, I hope won't be as foolish. Now here's the good news: plastic surgeon homework is pretty easy. It's not calculus, people. Even a chimp—who's wanted to deal with her facial hair for years—could do the research. And what's a little legwork, if you're going to have face work?

## How to Find That Great Plastic Surgeon or Dermatologist

Start by asking everyone you know. And by "everyone," I mean:

- **Your hair stylist.** He sees the hidden scars in hairlines and behind the ears day after day. He looks down blouses for hours, even though he's got absolutely no interest. He's seen good boob jobs and lousy ones. Believe me, he's an expert on who does great work and who doesn't. And I'll bet you he can rattle off names and phone numbers.

- **Your primary-care doctor, or gynecologist.** He sees it all, he's heard all the horror stories, seen all the successes. But beware if he recommends himself to do your Restylane or other injections. Always go with a specialist!

- **Friends and acquaintances.** They might be a close or just a casual friend. You might feel a tad uncomfortable going up to her at a party, pointing at her boobs, and asking where she got 'em. But if she has implants, I promise you, she's not a shy type, and would probably drop her halter to let you feel them while singing the praises of her surgeon. If so, check out her scars. Take the opportunities when they come.* Most women are happy and proud to share. Be aware that women will tell you who did their breasts, while looking at you through newly lifted eyes, *totally* denying they've done anything to their face.

- **Google.** For women who simply cannot bring themselves to get referrals from people, the Internet is your friend! Use it as often as your vibrator. Do Google searches (for example, "best plastic surgeons in NYC" or "best plastic surgeons in Wichita"). A lot of regional magazines do annual roundups on the best doctors in the area, so try a search for the article in the local publication's website. Also, go to one of my favorite resources—www.plasticsurgery.org—to do a search of surgeons in your zip code, along with a coding system of recommendations and links to individual doctor's websites.

---

*This is also a great way to find a lesbian lover.

# How to Crack a Tough Nut

Many women have a secret cosmetic surgery life. You know the type: Everyone knows she's having work done, but she refuses to admit it. You might even know a woman who claims her perfect skin is due to a vacation on the island of St. Bart's, when it was actually St. Bart's Medical Center. Robert Redford had a face lift but said he was just rested. That's partially true. He fell asleep on the operating table.

If a woman is out of the plastic surgery closet, you could ask her for her doctor's name. But if she's not, you can't. What you can do, however, is be circumspect, and try these strategies.

**Give to get.** Make like you have no idea she's been peeled/lifted/Botoxed, and confide to her that you fantasize about having skin just like hers. Go on and on about how much you hate your skin. Lay it on thick. She'll surely give you a referral, probably couched ("a friend of mine told me about Doctor X").

**Go passive-aggressive.** By that, I mean send an email. I get a hundred spam emails a day asking if my erections are as hard as they used to be (and, thanks to Viagra, I'm proud to report that they are). Or if I'd like to join the Hoodia revolution. Why can't you shoot off a note that reads, "Hello! How are you? I'm fine, thanks. Actually, I'm not fine. I have a hateful bump on my nose that I desperately want to change. I've been casting a wide net, asking for referrals, and since you're so together and polished, I thought you might have a friend who can give me the name of a great doctor."

She'll spill. Oh, yes, she will spill.

By the way, this formula (self-deprecation + flattery = putty in your hands) works on just about anyone, from a housekeeper to a federal court judge.

Once you have a short list of qualified doctors, narrow it down to three names. How to shrink an already selective list? With the precision of a surgeon's scalpel. It's a buyer's market. Surgeons, even qualified, experienced types, are a dime a dozen. Remember, you are in control. You are The Decider, so first of all:

**Verify his qualifications.** What you're looking for is board certification in plastic surgery, or board certification in dermatology, depending on what you want done. Board certification in a specialty means the doctor has had years of training in that specialty. Just as you wouldn't go to a plastic surgeon for a heart transplant, you shouldn't go to a podiatrist for a nose job. Or a dermatologist for a nose job, for that matter.

To extract the blackheads on your nose, yes, run to Dr. Skin. But to have the skin on the nose peeled back like a grape, go to a surgeon who has shaved hundreds if not thousands of nasal humps.

To check a doc's board certification and specialty, go to www. abms.org, the website for the American Board of Medical Specialties. Once there, you have to register your email address and a password. It's really simple. I did it myself, without having to hire another assistant. Then, you follow prompts to enter your doctor's name. And there he should be. Board-certified as a specialist in plastic surgery, just like the diploma on his wall says. For further refinement, go to www.plasticsurgery.org, the website for the American Society of Plastic Surgeons. They list doctors who have specialties in plastic surgery, at least six years of training and experience in surgery, with three years specifically in plastic surgery, who are certified by the American Board of Plastic Surgery, who work out of an accredited facility (look for the American Association for Accreditation of Ambulatory Surgical Facilities' stamp of approval). It's as close to a comprehensive and complete credentials check as you can do online. Next,

**Visit the doctor's website.** I've got my own website (www.joan

rivers.com), and I take a lot of pride in its appearance and content. Keeping an updated blog and posting photos is the least I can do for my fans—well, fan. I expect a doctor to maintain a website as a service to potential customers. If he doesn't have one, or his website is cheesy and hard to navigate, forget it. In what other business is presentation more important? On his site, you need to find a nice gallery of "before" and "after" photos. Also, read some of the patient testimonials (often very touching; they might make you cry). Of course, check out the doctor's photo and feel free to judge him on *his* appearance. You've heard the expression, "Never trust a skinny chef." How about: "Never trust an ugly plastic surgeon," or "Never trust an acne-scarred dermatologist." Then:

**Call his office.** Who answers the phone? Is it a friendly, helpful person, or a disinterested snippy asswipe? If you wanted to deal with a rude, barely conscious robot, you'd seek out a saleslady at Chanel. At a doctor's office, you want to be treated with respect. Are you put on hold? Long enough to piss you off? Long enough to hang up? Or are you catered to, spoken kindly to, paid the proper attention? If you like them, make an appointment for a consultation. Some doctors charge for the initial office visit; most don't.

Last, you must meet the doctor face to face. Also important, you need to see his office and surgical facility. And his receptionist, as she'll be the one you'll be dealing with. And his nurses (likewise). In the waiting room, you'll get to talk to some of his patients, see how happy/unhappy they've been. Believe me, unhappy patients will be bursting to tell you their complaints. Often, in the waiting room, doctors have binders of before-and-after photos to flip through—an excellent way to pass time. His waiting room should also have comfortable, clean seating, current magazines, nicely arranged, and some soothing music piped in. You'll be spending a lot of time there. Why shouldn't every aspect of the experience be pleasant?

In your city, there are probably fifty doctors who would bare-knuckle fight for your business. You should expect and receive the best.

## Two Important Warnings

Warning #1: I beg you, do *not* be tempted by the classified ads in the newspaper, the type that screams, "Three-Area Lipo, No Money Down!" The low prices might catch your attention. But is hiring a surgeon the right time to go bargain hunting? As a plastic surgeon friend puts it, "Doctors know what they're worth, and they create a price list based on that." An expensive surgeon has the experience and results to back up his pricing. Listen to me! You get what you pay for in life, from shoes to surgeons. Inexpensive pumps fall apart in a season. A bargain boob job? In a year, you'll pay more to have the implants removed.

Cheap ends up expensive, and expensive ends up cheap.

Do not feel tempted to save a buck and go overseas to Asia or Eastern Europe for bargain-basement-priced plastic surgery. This new trend, called "surgery safaris," which combines a tourist vacation to, say, Thailand or Greece, with a nose job and breast lift, is a booming business of some $100 million a year. The problem(s) with having operations abroad: 1) there's no guarantee the doctor or hospital is up to standards, 2) you won't be able to go in for follow-up visits, and, the biggie, 3) if something goes wrong, like the account I read of a woman who went to a developing country for a face lift and came home with her ears behind her head, you will have to pay the full freight for a do-over (if possible) back home anyway.

For that matter, don't go for a bargain in the States, either. Say you go to an unqualified, inexpensive surgeon, and wind up with a nose job that looks like the roll of pennies you used to pay for it. You'll have to have it corrected with another surgery, and wind up paying more than you would have had you gone to the expensive surgeon in the first place.

Or, as my old Irish* grandmother used to say, "Buy well, weep once."

Warning #2: Get ready for sticker shock. The flat belly of your dreams? It may cost you the price of a renovated bathroom. A breast reduction? That's your anniversary vacation in Paris. A year of Botox Cosmetic? Good-bye Hamptons rental. It's about priorities. Do you want a new face or a new patio? Even if you've got a two-hour commute, you've got a twenty-four-hour face.

As I've always said, take your pick: Is it better to have a new face getting out of an old car, or an old face getting out of a new car? If you're hankering for a change, put off your vacation and renew your lease on the clunker. Tolerate the hardwater stains on the tub for a bit longer, and get that cosmetic procedure.

Some other quick cautions about picking a doctor. Run the other way if:

- He carries a copy of *Plastic Surgery for Dummies* under his arm.
- His diploma is from Jugs "R" Us Academy.
- He jokes that his receptionist is his "patients' spare parts."
- His name is Dr. Frankenstein.
- Or Dr. Kevorkian.
- He's so cocky about his work, he signs his name on all his patients' rear ends.
- He has a sub-specialty in taxidermy.

## The In-Office Consultation

The great architect Mies van der Rohe said, "God is in the details." And he was right. Every detail of your consultation is relevant. Be

---

*Irish, Jewish—don't quibble. They both end in "ish."

as nitpicky as you wish. I gave this instruction to a friend who was looking for a plastic surgeon and sent her to three offices for consultations. Her objective was to judge each doctor by the Rule of Small Things. As it turned out, paying attention to detail made her decision much easier. I'll just let her tell it . . .

## Doctor #1: We'll Call Him Dr. Roger

"I got Dr. Roger's name from my primary-care physician. I confirmed his credentials at the websites Joan gave me. Dr. Roger's office was only a few blocks from my apartment in Brooklyn Heights, so he got points for convenience. When I called for an appointment, the receptionist put me on hold twice. I took it as a sign he was in demand, which had to be a good thing."

"On the day of the appointment, I was pretty nervous. I'd been fantasizing about a breast reduction/tummy tuck for years. I probably never would have made the appointment if it weren't for Joan asking me to do this experiment. I was dying of curiosity about what Dr. Roger would say. I half hoped he'd take one look at my belly and say, 'You're fine. You don't need any work.' I soon came to learn, in my week of visiting plastic surgeons, that most of them are not in the business of sending you home.

"Anyway, I arrived on time at Dr. Roger's office. The receptionist was cute, young. I asked if she'd had any work done by Dr. Roger, and she said no. I asked if she had books of before-and-after photos I could look at, and she said Dr. Roger didn't like to show pictures to clients because everyone was different, and comparisons were meaningless. I then sat and waited twenty minutes to be called in to see the doctor, which kind of annoyed me as I was his first appointment of the day. Since Joan told me to be petty and demanding, I took to checking my watch aggressively and sighing loudly, but the receptionist turned up the volume on her iPod and ignored me.

"Finally, I was shown into Dr. Roger's office. Like the waiting room, it was clean but cold. Dr. Roger himself was decent-looking. Tall and slim, attractively put together, and nattily dressed. He didn't smile at all, though. And he seemed irked that I had a notepad and a list of questions. He suggested I hold off until after he'd examined me.

"Off we went into the exam room. He gave me a surgical gown. I undressed except for my panties. He returned, asked me to stand up in front of him—he was seated on a stool—and to open my robe. Yikes. I've never really felt a hundred percent comfortable naked with strange men, even doctors. If Dr. Roger sensed my nervousness, he did nothing to alleviate it. After looking at my boobs for a minute, he said, 'You don't need a breast reduction. You need a lift.' Using white surgical tape, he hoisted my left boob and affixed it to my upper chest. It was higher, and tighter. He said a lift and a small amount of lipo would make my boobs manageable. Since my complaint was their unwieldiness, the lift idea made sense. We were having this whole conversation with one breast taped up, and the other sagging halfway down my chest.

"Then Dr. Roger asked me to lie down on the exam room table. He grabbed handfuls of my belly and called the upper abdominal load 'hard-pack fat,' which, although true, wasn't very nice. The lower abdominal pouch, he said, was 'loose skin left over from pregnancy. You'll never get rid of it, even if you lost a lot of weight.' He recommended a full tummy tuck, with lipo of the love handles (which I hadn't even asked about). I got dressed and met him back in his office.

"By now, the fantasy of getting surgery had already turned into a clinical reality. Dr. Roger's manner wasn't comforting, or encouraging. In his office, he leaned back in his chair and dispassionately explained the recovery for each procedure. He avoided a description of the operation itself, even though I asked. Did he think I couldn't handle it? For the breast lift, he quoted $9,000. For the tummy tuck: $12,500. For both at once: $20,000. I must have looked shocked.

He said, 'I don't do bargain surgery. For that price, you get the best of everything. You'll be well-medicated.' So he gives expensive drugs? Should that sell me? I felt vaguely offended and demoralized. Dr. Roger came off rather cocky about his skills. But if he was so sure of himself, why didn't he show before-and-after photos? I told him it was a lot to think about, thanked him, and left. He'd spent a total of thirty minutes with me. Counting the wait, I'd been there just under an hour. The receptionist said she'd call in a few days to follow up.

"I said, 'Don't call me; I'll call you.' "

## Doctor #2: We'll Call Him Dr. Josh

"I found Dr. Josh by doing a zip code search on www.plasticsurgery. org. All the doctors in this search engine are board-certified specialists with accredited facilities. Dr. Josh had a blue dot next to his name, meaning he was a standout. I was very impressed by Dr. Josh's website, which included an extensive before-and-after gallery, and by his office's Central Park West address. His receptionist was beyond friendly when I called. As promised, she emailed me downloadable video programs about tummy tucks and breast reductions. The videos lasted about twenty-five minutes each and detailed the operations in graphic—but not gnarly—detail. Highly instructive! So far, so good! I couldn't wait to tell Joan.

"I arrived at my appointment fifteen minutes early and expected to twiddle my thumbs. That wouldn't have been terrible, actually. The waiting room had plush couches and tons of reading material, including current issues of intelligent magazines. Just as I was getting comfortable, I was called into the exam room. No waiting! In the room, a nurse gave me a gown and paper panties. She told me Dr. Josh had done her nose, her chin, and her tummy tuck. On her birthday, she was going to get thigh lipo. The nose job looked pretty good. And her belly was flat, as far as I could tell. The exam room, like the waiting room, was beautiful, fully loaded with equipment and magazines, and had a big leather chair in lieu of a cold exam table.

"Dr. Josh arrived promptly and read my paperwork. He was a compact guy, nicely dressed and neatly shaved. Instead of asking about my boobs and belly, his first question was, 'You're a writer? What kind of stuff?' And then we talked about my career and our favorite authors. He acted like he had all day to kibitz with me. After ten minutes, he smoothly transitioned into shop talk. 'As a novelist, you have flexible hours. That's good for your recovery. So let's have a look at your breasts.' I felt more comfortable showing my body to him. Unlike Dr. Roger, Dr. Josh used tools to measure me. A caliper and measuring tape. He took notes and asked me what my vision was for my breasts. He suggested a lift with minor reduction, just as Dr. Roger had. For the belly, he took more measurements and recommended a full tummy tuck with love handle lipo. He spent a total of forty-five minutes with me.

"He left. I dressed, and the receptionist came back in with three printouts breaking down the costs of just a breast lift ($8,500), just a tummy tuck ($9,000), and both at once ($14,500). She handed each sheet to me, explained what was on it, and asked me to sign a copy to keep in my file should I go ahead with surgery. She spent another fifteen minutes talking to me about how she got from thinking about having surgery to actually doing it—a giant step, I was realizing.

"I left feeling comforted and catered to. If I were to go ahead with the operations, I was confident I'd be well cared for by Dr. Josh and his staff. I also liked his prices."

## Doctor #3: We'll Call Him Dr. Mark

"Just for variety, I thought I'd see a guy who advertised in the local newspaper classified section. I called his office and spoke to his

receptionist. She seemed a bit ditzy, but sweet. I told her I was interested in a tummy tuck and breast reduction. She made the appointment and called twice to confirm.

"I showed up on time, filled out the forms. Dr. Mark's office was
a mess. His receptionist apologized and said they were in the process of moving. I sympathized. Moving is never fun. But having to
sit amongst half-packed boxes and garbage bags didn't fill me with
confidence in Dr. Mark. If he were professional about it, he would
have rented a transitional space. I was nervous.

"A chubby, older guy in a rumpled shirt with the sleeves slop-
pily rolled up found me in the cluttered waiting area and introduced
himself. This was Dr. Mark? Points off for personal appearance. I followed him to the exam room. He told me he was a retired ob/gyn
surgeon. 'I spent thirty years doing hysterectomies and Caesarians.
So many women came to me after their pregnancies for referrals to
plastic surgeons to get rid of their bellies, I figured, why not learn
how to do tummy tucks myself?' he said.

"I asked, 'So you're not board certified in plastic surgery?'

"He said, 'I am board certified.'

" 'But not in plastic surgery?' I repeated. He shrugged it off. I remembered Joan's warning about doctors doing plastic surgery without obtaining a specialty in it.

"So we're in the exam room—which, disgustingly, had used
gloves and detritus on a tray nearby—and I showed him my belly.
He looked at it for ten seconds and then said I could lower my shirt.
'Don't you need to see my breasts?' I asked. He said he didn't work on
breasts but he knew a doctor who did. I distinctly remember telling
his receptionist about wanting a tummy tuck *and* a breast reduction.
A bait and switch?

"We went into his office. He had to move a box so I could sit
down. Dr. Mark said he'd done two 'girls' whose bellies looked like
mine recently, and he pulled up their before-and-after photos on his
website. This part of the presentation was impressive. He had loads

of pictures, from many angles, including some graphic pictures from the actual operations.

"Dr. Mark said I'd need upper abdomen lipo, and a mini tuck for the lower abdomen. My belly button wouldn't need to be relocated—a different recommendation than Dr. Roger and Dr. Josh, both specialists in plastic surgery. Next, Dr. Mark recited a speech about the wonders of liposuction and how a tummy tuck would change my life, how a lot of women used it as a jumping-off point to eating right and exercising. Meanwhile, he hadn't asked me a thing about my lifestyle and health. As he babbled on, at one point, he glanced at his watch! The next thing he said was the most shocking, considering his credentials, office, and the rushed exam. For the mini tuck and lipo, he wanted $10,000! Less surgery than either Dr. Roger or Dr. Josh, and more money. I thanked him and left. I'd been there for a total of twenty-five minutes.

"When and if I move forward, I'll go with Dr. Josh. He was superior in every regard. He was the only doctor who talked to me like a person. He and his staff seemed to understand a patient's need to feel comforted and assured that the process would run smoothly. Interestingly, the doctor with the nicest office was charging the least."

My friend now understood the value of face-to-face meetings with potential doctors. At the end of the day, every woman has to pick a doctor she likes on a personal level. I'm not impressed by a doctor who's brilliant but a bastard. You need to make a human connection, to believe he sees you as more than a piece of meat with a price tag. Silly as it sounds, I've always believed that a doctor will take better care of you if he likes you, and you'll be able to express your desires more clearly if you like him.

# The Ultimate Litmus Test on Choosing a Doctor

Even after your round of consultations, you might still be on the fence about making a choice. A great litmus test is the doctor's collection of before-and-after photos. Besides the vicarious fun of looking at the breasts and noses of complete strangers and comparing yourself to them (as in, "I'm not nearly as bad as her," and "Look at the size of those flapjacks!"), before-and-after pix tell you oodles about your prospective doctor. His handiwork, his aesthetics, how many procedures he's done. I like to go to a doctor's office and find a huge binder of photos, organized by procedure, in the waiting room. It's amazing to see the incredible diversity of the human form. And there are some great clues to pick up on your doctor skills if you look carefully. For example, watch out if:

1. **Every patient has Halle Berry's nose,** as if the doctor makes body parts from a mold and glues them on every patient. Now, Halle Berry has a gorgeous nose. But it might not work on your face. The doc's photos should show that he pays attention to the needs of each individual patient. In a word, you want to see noses that "go."

2. **Make sure you see visible improvement.** Subtlety is good. But if you're spending all that money and time in recovery, you want to see results. There's a famous doctor in Los Angeles who made such subtle changes, it was a joke that he had to do everyone twice. "Conservative change" is great. After a good face lift, you should look better, brighter, more rested, but still look like you. However, there is a big different between subtle and "no difference." The point of having plastic surgery is to see *improvement*. If the patient looks fifty years old in the "before" shot, and forty-nine years old in the "after," that is not a good sign.

3.  **All of the photos appear to be the same handful of patients.** It's a major red flag if you don't see a big range of patients and procedures. Seeing the same woman over and over again (on page 1, her eye lift; page 5, her nose job; page 10, her lip augmentation) makes me wonder how much experience the surgeon has—or doesn't have. Since the choice is yours, go with a doctor who's helped hundreds of women.

## Doctors Are the New Lawyers?

Used to be, a doctor was considered to be the most honest and trustworthy member of society. My father was a doctor from the old school. He cared about his patients; he worried about them; he actually knew their names and histories, so it pains me to say the sad truth: *Some unscrupulous quacks will do anything for money.*

Cosmetic surgeries and procedures like Botox Cosmetic, collagen, and Restylane injections are very lucrative. The bad apples see an opportunity for easy money, and they take it. They'll lie, swindle, and sweet-talk you for your business. They'll claim to be board certified but won't say in what specialty.

One friend of mine heard of a proctologist who was performing face lifts! Although, for some people, having a face that looks like an ass would be an improvement. One of his patients got a lift so extreme, every time she said, "Hello," people thought she farted.

"The biggest issue today in this business is individuals who call themselves cosmetic surgeons without getting adequate training," said Robert Singer, M.D., past president of the American Society of Aesthetic Plastic Surgery, past chairman for the American Society of Plastic Surgery, and current president of the American Association for Accreditation of Ambulatory Surgical Facilities Education Foundation. He's also a surgeon with thirty years of experience at his clinic in San Diego. "Don't be fooled by 'cosmetic.' Anyone can call himself or herself a 'cosmetic surgeon,' having taken a one-week course on liposuction. Even less invasive procedures like fillers and peels have real risks that require the judgment and experience that only board certification in plastic surgery can provide." Singer has made it his mission to encourage patients to educate themselves about procedures and doctors. He wants to make his industry as safe and assessable as possible. For every great doctor out there, there's a quack with a shingle and a buzz-saw.

Don't believe Dr. Singer? Then believe me. I've got stories . . .

## Horror Stories

If you don't believe that picking a skilled, certified, trustworthy doctor is a critically important decision, I've got three words for you: Kanye West's mother.

**Horror story #1:** Donda West dreamed of a flat belly and perky boobs—and who doesn't? She sought out a doctor who could do a tummy tuck, breast reduction, breast implants, and liposuction. Problem was, Donda West was obese (5 feet, 2 inches and 188 pounds), had high blood pressure, and a cardiac artery blockage. By multiple accounts, Donda was turned away by, allegedly, at least two reputable doctors who pre-screen potential patients for health conditions that rule out elective surgery.

Enter Jan Adams, M.D., a surgeon who'd appeared on *Oprah, Extra*, and his own reality-based TV show about his life as a California plastic surgeon. Despite Donda's pre-existing conditions, Adams was willing to do the five-and-a-half-hour surgery on her. A day later, West was dead. Cause of death? According to published reports, her bad heart couldn't handle the stress of surgery.

In the days after her death, more information was revealed about Jan Adams, M.D. Turned out, he *wasn't* board certified in plastic surgery. Adams did have a certification in "general" surgery, which, according to California law, means a doctor can do plastic surgery. But it doesn't guarantee the doctor has been adequately trained. It also came to light that Adams had a nasty DUI habit. He was arrested—twice— for drunk driving. He'd been found guilty of malpractice—twice— and had to pay huge payouts. Although there was no evidence Adams botched the surgery on West, the big question is: Should he have done the surgery in the first place?

The moral of this story: Just as any reputable doctor pre-screens patients to make sure they're viable for surgery, *every patient should pre-screen her doctor to make sure he's viable to operate.* If Donda had done minimal investigation on Adams, she might be alive today. Last I read of Adams, he'd left the West Coast and now practices in Palm Beach, Florida. This is a good thing, since the people there are so old, most of his patients are already dead.

**Horror story #2:** Totie Fields, the huge comedienne—in many ways—of the 1960s and '70s, searched and searched for a doctor to get a face lift. This was thirty-five years ago. Face lifts have come a long way, but even in that day, no doctor worth his golf balls should have agreed to operate on her: Totie had diabetes and a heart condition. Eventually, she found a doctor who told her of the risks. But Totie insisted, and, finally, he gave in. The surgery caused a blood clot to lodge in her leg, which had to be amputated above the knee. And you know what she did? She sued the doctor! Was she right to do this? Some people feel the answer should be "yes." It was the surgeon's responsibility as a good doctor never to have let her walk through the door of the operating room. Totie died two years later, after having a few heart attacks that might have been accelerated by the trauma of amputation.

In our list of perils, so far we have death and dismemberment. Now let's add permanent pain.

**Horror story #3:** Ten years ago, a friend of mine got liposuction from a doctor she met at a cocktail party. They hit it off, and she made an appointment with him the very next day for major liposuction on her waist. The doctor went in too deep, and she's had pain in the spot ever since. It was only later after the damage was done that she found out he had a bad reputation among other doctors.

Then there are scars that won't heal properly.

**Horror story #4:** A decorator friend of mine got an acid peel in return for helping to redo the doctor's wife's living room. The doctor applied too much solution. It took months for her skin to recover, and it never looked normal again. She was so eager to get the procedure on the cheap; she trusted anyone in a white lab coat.

She should have looked on the lab coat's pocket and seen the emblem reading "Howard Johnson's."

**Horror story #5:** A friend, who's also a plastic surgeon, told me the story of a famous male movie star who went on vacation in South America and got so hammered at a party that he was convinced by a "surgeon" to let him work on his face that very night. When the actor woke up, the skin of his face had been severely lifted.

His lift was so high, he could see behind himself.

The star had to put his career on hold for two years, stay out of the public eye, until he had the problem fixed (not nearly enough).

**One more horror story, #6 (I know, six of them is a lot to take):** Priscilla Presley. Did you see her on "Dancing with the Stars"? More like Dancing with Madame Tussaud's Wax Figure.

In 2003, Presley fell under the influence of a "gigolo" (hey, TMZ said it first, not me), an Argentinean physician named Daniel Serrano. Serrano arrived in Hollywood and immediately started touting his miracle wrinkle eraser as God's gift to women.

I was immediately suspicious, since we all know God's gift to women is the vibrator.

The stuff in his syringe, what he called "better than Botox," was a low-grade silicone used to lubricate auto parts in Argentina, and most definitely *not* FDA approved for use in a human body. Can you imagine having your face pumped with the same stuff that kept Evita's 1939 Packard zipping through the streets of Buenos Aires?

Among Serrano's alleged clients were Larry King's wife, Shawn, and Lionel Richie's wife, Diane. They'd round up their friends for a Serrano lube job party, where he'd inject his "miracle" for $500 a shot. He quickly became known as Dr. Jiffy Lube. Eventually, he was arrested for illegally importing his poison, and served fifteen months in prison. A week after his release in 2008, he was arrested again by immigration officials who will most likely deport him.

It's tragic, how a gorgeous woman like Priscilla Presley can be scammed.* Reportedly, she's having corrective surgery to get the silicone out. Good luck to her.

And you? You won't need luck. You'll have referrals, credential checks, office consultations, among other research, to rely on. When it comes to choosing a doctor, luck has got nothing to do with it.

## Black Balls

I'm not talking about Billy Dee Williams or a Heidi Klum sex toy! I'm talking about disqualifying factors for plastic surgery. There are a lot. Here's a pretty good list of the health factors that would give any reputable surgeon SERIOUS pause.

- high blood pressure
- heart disease
- heart valve disorders
- diabetes
- smoking
- drug addiction
- alcoholism
- pulmonary disease
- anemia

- bleeding disorders
- hepatitis
- HIV-AIDS
- multiple sclerosis
- lupus
- arthritis
- scleroderma
- anorexia
- obesity

*Then again, she's a Scientologist.

These are just the physical reasons not to operate. Any patient who is emotionally unstable or mentally not-all-there should be shown the door by a doctor—and I don't mean the door to the operating room.

Bottom line: If you're high-risk, and go ahead with surgery anyway, you might not live to regret it. If three doctors tell you "no," don't go looking for a fourth.

## ( Two )

# **Botox,** Baby!

Joan had to begin somewhere so, after meeting a visiting California Barbie from next door, all she could focus on was the girl's perfectly smooth cappuccino-colored skin. How could someone be so smooth and tan, Joan thought to herself?

Joan noticed immediately, when she got home, that her own forehead had more lines on it than Lindsay Lohan's coffee table. And these weren't just fine lines, like the lines between whether or not Michael Jackson is a man/woman or black/white. The lines were deep and needed to be removed before they got any deeper. Joan knew something had to be done if she hoped to find a boyfriend, but only, as she insisted, if it did not involve doctors and needles. Joan had read that Botox sometimes left women with frozen looks on their faces, so she immediately booked a trip to the Arctic Circle and checked in to a budget igloo with its own ice machine. She hardly had time to unpack her snowsuit when brand-new lines started appearing on her forehead, thanks to annoying little things about the tundra like frostbite,

*gangrene, and a scarcity of kosher whale blubber. Joan jumped on the next*
*cargo plane home and, once she fully thawed out, called a dermatologist*
*and booked an appointment for Botox injections.*

A dermatologist once told me about the four Rs of facial rejuvenation: Relax, Refill, Resurface, and Redrape.

Refill is about injectable fillers, like Restylane. Resurface refers to various techniques to smooth the texture and tone of the skin. Redrape is the big guns of surgical lifts.

This chapter is about the first R: Relaxing your face with Botox Cosmetic injections. It's not only number one in the dermatologist's category system. It's number one among beauty seekers, and I mean huge. As big as Russell Crowe's ego. In 2007, 4.6 *million* Americans had Botox Cosmetic treatments.

The rest, unfortunately, still look like Bea Arthur.

The massive appeal? Botox Cosmetic (or, as it's commonly called, Botox) is not *like* magic. Truly, it *is* magic. A chemical miracle. Wave a syringe, and all your worries (or the appearance of them) disappear. Botox Cosmetic is, literally, an instant fix. And who doesn't love instant gratification? What is sexier and more beautiful than young, smooth skin? Men want to gaze into a woman's relaxed, clear, and smooth face, as if she hasn't a concern in the world, except how better to please him. He doesn't need to see her worries and anxieties and— worst of all—the proof of her irritation with him etched across her brow. A face that *appears* placid is alluring, reassuring, and sexy.

Who can forget the corpse of Anna Nicole Smith? The worried woman behind the unworried skin?

Well. Botox Cosmetic won't make your problems go away, but a smooth forehead is one less thing to worry about.

# Botox Basics

When I first saw the word "botulism," it was in screaming headlines about poison cans of soup. Some readers might remember the 1972 vichyssoisse botulism scare. One man died eating the poisoned Bon Vivant brand soup. His wife was hospitalized. A massive recall effectively put Bon Vivant out of business.

Botulinum toxin, the bacteria, was first discovered two hundred years ago, in Germany, when it grew on a rotten sausage. The word botulism is a version of the Latin *butulus*, which means sausage.

Rest assured, when you use Botox Cosmetic you won't be injecting sausage into your face. What you do behind closed doors is your own business. You'll be injecting a bacteria byproduct that grows on decaying sausage.

Chemically speaking, botulinum toxin is a protein. It's created by the bacteria *clostridium botulinum* that grows on bad meat. Like daisies, butterflies, and puppy dogs, it is one of God's creatures. For a long time, it was considered to be the Earth's Most Toxic Protein! or Worst Poison Found in Nature! Before doctors thought to inject it into people's faces to make them look pretty, the government tried to turn botulinum toxin into a WMD during the WWII era, calling the bomb project Agent X.* You could almost see the name Agent X used in a marketing campaign for a skin care line today.

Botox was the nickname for botulinum toxin type A. Only a minute percentage of the actual toxin goes into the syringe—hardly any, actually. Or, I should say, *just enough*. Humans got their first dose in the 1980s to treat eye twitching and crossed eyes. The stuff worked, and the practice of using Botox for optic disorders took hold. A husband and wife pair of doctors, Jean and Alastair Carruthers from Vancouver, realized that not only were the patients' eye conditions better,

---

*Had they dropped this bomb on the Soviet Union, there would have been prettier contestants in the Miss Moscow beauty pageant.

but they looked extremely well rested. No more lines between the eyebrows. Their crow's feet turned into angel whispers.

Faster than you can say "ten years younger," Allergan, a pharmaceutical company, started turning out Botox Cosmetic as a treatment for forehead wrinkles. In 1992, the FDA approved it. Since then, it has been injected into millions of faces all over the world.

FYI: "Botox" is the preparation of the drug used on eye twitches and other spasms of the face and neck. "Botox Cosmetic" is the preparation used to treat wrinkles. The most commonly injected areas for Botox Cosmetic are the horizontal forehead lines, the two vertical lines between the eyebrows (the elevens, as they say in England), and crow's feet.

## How It Works

Habitual facial movements cause wrinkles. Over time, the wrinkles become etched in your skin. What controls the muscles? Nerves. Facial nerves release neurotransmitter chemicals that signal muscles to move. Botox Cosmetic blocks the nerve from putting out the neurotransmitter acetylcholine. Without the chemical go-ahead, the facial muscles might as well be an inert steak on a slab. Without the chemical signal, the muscle is essentially paralyzed. It does not move. So if you have no muscle movement, you'll have—voilà!—no wrinkles. It takes about four months for your skin to break down the toxin and for acetylcholine to stage a comeback. The muscles will start moving again, and the wrinkles will slowly reappear.

However, one great thing about Botox Cosmetic is that the more you use it, the less you need to. If you keep the nerve chemical blocked for eighteen months by getting regular treatments, the muscles begin to atrophy. Any muscle that isn't used will weaken, and eventually, the muscles become so feeble, they won't contract much, even after the Botox Cosmetic wears off. When the wrinkles start to show up again, they're not as deep, and people can go longer between treatments.

## How It's Done

It's fast! And instant! The actual procedure takes minutes. After you've been shown into the examining room, the doctor (a dermatologist or plastic surgeon—don't even *think* of letting anyone less qualified stick needles in your face!) will do a quick check of your skin tone and facial wrinkles. You'll be asked to make some faces so he can see how and where you wrinkle. Your wrinkles will become the guidelines for where the doctor will target the Botox Cosmetic.

I asked Shilesh Iyer, M.D., a Yale- and Harvard-trained doctor at the New York Dermatology Group on Fifth Avenue, a diplomat of the American Board of Dermatology, and a fellow of the American Academy of Dermatology, American Society for Dermatologic Surgery, and American Society for Laser Medicine and Surgery, where he likes to inject the needle. "Muscles produce the wrinkle," he said, "so I ask patients to make faces to see how their muscles contract, not to find the wrinkles. Injections are made into the muscles, not into the wrinkles themselves. Any trained doctor knows the anatomy of facial muscles. That's why you have to see a doctor for Botox Cosmetic treatments."

The number of shots depends on the treatment area. Dr. Iyer said, "Usually, I do four or five shots across the forehead. For frown lines, three to five. Crow's feet, three shots on each side," he said. To treat larger areas, like the rings around the neck, he does more. "To relax the platysma muscles in the neck, I do two or three rows of five injections."

The depth of the shots also depends on the area. The eye and neck muscles are superficial, and the needle goes in shallowly. The muscles between your eyebrows are deeper, so the needle has to go in farther.

No matter how deep it goes in, the needle itself is tiny. "Most people are shocked by how easy it is to get a Botox Cosmetic treatment," said Dr. Iyer. "And, unfortunately, that's why so many untrained people are giving them."

Me? I go in for shots every six months or so. Most doctors will tell a patient the pain is minimal, but I think the injections hurt. They don't want to have to give you topical numbing cream because it takes fifteen minutes to take effect. They'd rather have you in, sit you down, load the syringe, bingo, bango, bongo, you're out of there. So either get a prescription for numbing cream and put it on yourself beforehand, or make good friends with the nurses and get them to give you some to apply while in the waiting room.

Results are almost immediate. You'll have to wait a few days to see the change, but by week's end, the Botox Cosmetic is in full effect. The creases are ironed out and will stay that way for four months. When the wrinkles start to reappear, you know when it's time for another treatment.

## Off-Label Use

Like nearly every drug on the market, doctors have figured out beneficial applications that have nothing to do with what the drug was originally used for or given FDA approval for. Like women taking Viagra. Or spraying Windex on pimples.

Botox Cosmetic, you should know, has only one officially sanctioned application—to get rid of frown lines caused by the glabellar muscles between the eyebrows.

Any other use of Botox Cosmetic is "off-label." That includes using it on crow's feet, horizontal forehead lines, and the hateful rings around your neck. If you get such treatments, you're not breaking the law, and you won't be carted off to jail, nor will your doctor. Every doctor I spoke to said Botox Cosmetic is just as safe and effective in the crow's feet as it is between the eyebrows, so don't ask me why the

FDA is so damn picky about where you can and cannot shoot botulinum toxin in your face.

I've also heard of many dermatologists injecting Botox Cosmetic into women's armpits in June to prevent unsightly sweating all summer long. No, I'm serious!

As I've explained, Botox Cosmetic is the only preparation used to treat wrinkles. Another formula, Botox, has a higher percentage of the toxin, and is FDA-approved to treat eye disorders like twitching, crossed, and wandering eye, and spasms in the neck and back. It's also used to stop excessive sweating in the palms. Migraine sufferers await results of a study currently underway to ease their symptoms with Botox. There are other studies testing Botox on neurological disorders like epilepsy and cerebral palsy. We'll see how huge a drug it becomes over the next several years.

For all we know, it could be the miracle drug of the twenty-first century.

Then again, if the toxin were good for nothing more than making the world a prettier place, as far as I'm concerned, it would still win a spot in the Bacteria Hall of Fame.

## So, What's This Gonna Cost Me?

According to the American Society of Aesthetic Plastic Surgery, the national average for a Botox Cosmetic treatment is $382 a syringe. Depending on where you live, you will pay more than $382 per syringe. I came across a Botox Cosmetic price map that divided America into zones. Guess which region was the most expensive? The Northeast, thanks to New York City, where the average price was $510/syringe. The next priciest region was the Southeast, with its aging population in Florida, which had an average of $502. Next came the Southwest, and its millions of aging Texas debutantes. The average fee there was $382. Next, the Midwest, with an average fee of $377. And, the least expensive region? The West, from Colorado to California. You can get

Botox Cosmetic for a very reasonable $369 in the region. I can assure you, however, if you want to pay New York or Palm Beach prices in Los Angeles, you will NOT have a hard time finding someone to take your money.

Dr. Iyer told me that one syringe is all you'll need for a face, even if you treated a couple of areas. Be wary of a doctor who tries to sell you half a syringe worth. He might be trying to finish off what was left over from his last patient.

## Remind Me Again, Why Do I Want to Do This?

The biggest reasons we all love Botox Cosmetic?

**It Works.** As one doctor friend, the wonderful, amazing Pat Wexler, told me recently, "You know why there are so many different fillers, peels, and laser treatments on the market? Because none of them are perfect, or work on every person all the time. If there was one foolproof laser or one amazing filler, it would become the gold standard, and the others would fade away. *Botox Cosmetic is the gold standard.* It works every time, on every body. The only potential danger is the person holding the needle. If you have a skilled and experienced doctor doing the injections, you will love the results."

**It gives you an *air de mystère*.** Since you were a little girl, you admired the mysterious beauty of Greta Garbo. Well, with an un-lined face and limited expressiveness, you, too, can be Garboesque, opaque and inscrutable, letting only the gleam of your eyes give a hint of your true feelings. Those who ordinarily wear their hearts on their sleeves can now take comfort in keeping some emotional privacy for a change. No one needs to see every tiny feeling flit across your face. Botox Cosmetic is a guaranteed way to keep 'em guessing.

**Promise in a needle.** Max Factor famously said that makeup was hope in a jar. He certainly ran with that notion and created an empire. Botox Cosmetic is more than hope in a needle. It's a promise that you can stay fresh and beautiful, safely and quickly (if not so cheaply).

Wrinkles add years to your face, and Botox Cosmetic takes them right off. *You are as young as you look.* Botox Cosmetic might not be spouting from the fountain of youth . . . actually, it IS spouting from the fountain of youth! And it's yours for the taking.

## What's the Worst That Could Happen?

Okay, about the risks:

Maybe, after a treatment, you might get a wee **headache**. Or **nausea. Flu-ish symptoms**. A splotch of **redness** where the needle went in, or a twinge of **pain**. Worst case, you could get some temporary **eyelid droopage** or general **weakness in the eye area**. Here are the potential problems:

**Kabuki mask syndrome.** Not a medical condition. Just your average, everyday creep show example of too much of a good thing. Some people do not understand the meaning of the word "moderation." Too much Botox Cosmetic in too many areas on one face = a frozen mask. It all depends on how much the doctor puts in. If you're worried about looking like a mummy, tell your doctor about your fears. He'll err on the side of caution and use small amounts. Wait a week and, if you want more, go back.

Just go to Beverly Hills. I have not seen that many frozen faces since the Donner Party.

**Communication breakdown.** You might have trouble communicating basic human emotions non-verbally.

Your husband comes home and announces he just got a huge raise at work. Then he says, "Why aren't you smiling?" You say, "I *am* smiling."

Granted, most people don't get Botox Cosmetic around the mouth and chin, not if they need to eat to live (unlike Victoria Beckham).

Even if you can move your face (and you should be able to), the expressiveness of your eyes and forehead will be slightly downplayed.

It's a choice.

Personally, I'd rather look younger and *feel* happy than look older and be depressed. Just get used to declaring your emotions.

"I'm thrilled!"

"I'm sad!"

"I'm sexually frustrated and have been for ten years!"

**Botox brow.** Again, this is a problem of too much of a good thing. If you over-juiced your forehead muscles, your eyebrows might get an arched appearance. A witchy, "The Joker" style forehead is called Botox brow.

Just scale back on your next treatment.

**The danger of easy access.** Do not be tempted to go to Botox Cosmetic parties where women sit around someone's living room as a "nurse" or "technician" makes the rounds with a loaded syringe. How can you be sure the needler has any training? Or that he or she knows how to handle the toxin? (For instance, it should be stored cold.) There's no guarantee that it's Botox Cosmetic in the syringe. It could be Kool-Aid, saline, or antifreeze, for all you know.

If I were invited to a mud mask party, fine. Go. Have your fun. But do not, do not, do NOT attend a Botox Cosmetic party, unless it's given by a dermatologist or plastic surgeon, at his office, during regular business hours.

**Myth risks.** Two reports came out recently that raised doubts about the safety of botulinum toxin type A: Both reports turned out to be nothing as far as Botox Cosmetic is concerned. But to cover all the bases, here's what was said:

**Report #1:** An Italian study found that Botox injected on one side of a rat's brain traveled across to the other. Also, that Botox injected into rat whiskers wound up in their brains. When this study was published in April 2008, worldwide panic ensued. Botox causes brain damage! Alzheimer's! Dementia!

Everyone relax! The purified stuff the Italian scientists injected was NOT the preparation used for wrinkles. Scientists concluded that there wasn't a legitimate comparison between the two different concentrations of botulinum toxin type A. Botox Cosmetic has been used for almost two decades as a wrinkle treatment, without any neurological or brain disorders occurring.

**Report #2:** In early 2008, a watchdog group called Public Citizen alerted the FDA of sixteen Botox-related deaths, claiming the toxin traveled from the treatment site to other body parts, causing muscle weakness, and problems swallowing and breathing.

The dead were, tragically, children getting off-label high doses of the drug to treat cerebral palsy. None of them were Botox Cosmetic patients.

Public Citizen wants to have warning labels put on Botox Cosmetic packaging. At this writing, the FDA is investigating whether a warning label is justified. Meanwhile, the percentage of people who have had any adverse reaction to Botox Cosmetic is too tiny to calculate. Millions do it. In the report by Public Citizen, one woman was hospitalized after getting a treatment, but Botox Cosmetic wasn't necessarily the cause.

If you have any doubts, talk to your doctor. Afterward, should you have lingering worries, forget about the treatment. All cosmetic intervention is *voluntary*.* If you're not excited to do it, then don't!

## Don't Cry Over Spilled Ink

Piercing and tattooing, I have to say, are not for me. The only needles I want touching my skin are full of Botox Cosmetic.

Not that I haven't been tempted to try the trends once. I put in a nipple ring, but my boobs had dropped so low that it kept getting snagged on the living room carpet, so I had to take it out.

Generally, I think tattoos are for the young. When they get older, they

---

*But should have been mandatory for my cousin Bella.

fade and turn blue. Have you seen Cher's ass lately? It looks like she sat on a village of Smurfs.

According to a recent article in *Psychology Today* (what? you think I only read *People* and *Vogue*?), people with tattoos and piercings are assumed by others to be whores, drunks, and druggies.

But enough about Courtney Love.

The researchers didn't use my choice of words, but they might as well have. Tattoos, despite going mainstream, still suggest a rock-and-roll attitude, a biker-chick-ness, a permissive and promiscuous lifestyle. Like I said, body art is your personal advertisement.

Regardless of the design, a tattoo and piercing send the message "I'll Do You for Beer!"

The article in *Psychology Today* also said that those with body art are, actually, no sluttier and lushier than anyone else. (Except, of course, Paris Hilton.)

You might be a teetotaling virgin (*riiight*), but you thought getting a tattoo or nose ring would give you a cool, modern vibe. Now, instead of giving you street cred, you're getting hit on by ex-cons and Hell's Angels. Perhaps looking edgy is not as much fun as you hoped.

So what happens when the spiky and inky decide, after all, they'd rather not have the tongue stud or tramp stamp? What do they do to get rid of tats and holes?

Glad you asked. Here's a basic primer on unloading body art:

**Piercing closure.** You will never have an easier time correcting a mistake. To close a piercing hole, the first step is to remove the hardware.

Second step, wait.

The hole, depending on placement, will start to seal immediately. Tongues close faster than the ear. If you've had a piercing for a long time, the hole will take longer to close up. But, rest assured, every unused hole will eventually seal itself up.

(I don't even need to say it, but I will: VAGINA!)

Use it or lose it, as they say. With a closed piercing, you'll have a small scar where the hole used to be, and possibly some scar tissue (a bump under the skin). That's all. Life goes on.

**Tattoo erasure.** Tat removal used to involve sanding away multiple layers of skin or cutting away the entire chunk of skin and suturing back together what's left. Not fun. Today, tattoo removal via laser isn't quite as extreme. It hurts a bit—like repeatedly snapping a rubber band on your skin—but probably not as much as getting the tattoo did in the first place.*

It is, however, painful in a monetary sense. The price for erasure depends on the size of the tattoo in question. A little ink spot of a heart on a string might be erased for $300. A bicep-long mermaid riding a donkey might cost $1,000. A reproduction of Picasso's *Guernica* on your back might run you as much as, oh, say, $5,000 to eradicate.

As you know, the tattoo itself is colored ink permanently injected into the dermis, the deep layer of skin. To break up the ink, a dermatologist will use a hand-held laser to flash concentrated pulses of light on your tattoo. The light will penetrate into the dermis, where it's absorbed by the ink's pigment. The laser light then vaporizes and breaks up the color. The fragments of pigment are flushed from the body by your immune system. Each color requires a different wavelength of laser light. Black absorbs all laser light, so it's easiest to get rid of. Now, the truly scary part. You might need up to ten sessions, four to six weeks apart. The stamp will fade a little bit more each session. It could take up to a year to completely eradicate the tat you got impulsively one night when you were out on the town.

So next time you feel the urge to visit Tijuana, try temporary tattoos. My eight-year-old grandson loves them. You can get ink transfer designs for grownups that last a few days, and come off by dabbing with alcohol on a cotton ball. You can walk on the wild side for a naughty night, without having to stay there.

*Although you were probably so drunk, you don't remember.

**One more tiny downside.** Except the possibility of loving it too much. You can go back to work five minutes after a treatment. You could go dancing that night. The only warning you'll get from your injector is to drink in moderation for the week before and after treatment and to stay out of the sun, which is good advice regardless, and not to lie down for four hours after a treatment.

## Celeb Botox Ticker

Just assume that every star over thirty on TV and in movies is using Botox Cosmetic, and your assumption is probably right. Plastic surgeon Anthony Youn, M.D., wrote on his funny Celebrity Cosmetic Surgery blog that the injections are so common in Hollywood, he notices when stars *don't* use Botox Cosmetic far more than when they do.

**Nicole Kidman** has been kicked around the block about her overuse, which showed on her frozen forehead and arched eyebrow. Then, in photos taken while she was pregnant, her forehead lines were suddenly visible and her eyebrows were straighter. The contrast—on the juice, off the juice—was obvious.*

**Vanessa Williams** has been a vocal supporter and user. She's told Barbara Walters that Botox Cosmetic is a "miracle" and that every woman she knows uses it. If you look at photos of her, you see that her forehead is unlined, but she does allow herself to have some crow's feet. The overall effect is of a woman who looks her years, but is fresh, awake, and happy. She should be! She's gorgeous!

**Teri Hatcher** isn't exactly "Desperate," either. She's admitted to using Botox Cosmetic, then she said she was against it. It seems she can't make up her mind—the one behind her suspiciously smooth forehead.

*Since we have gone to press, rumor has it that Nicole has hired a young Guatemalan woman to smile for her.

**Virginia Madsen** told interviewers that she used the injections to get rid of the vertical lines between her eyebrows, and, the next thing you know, she landed a hot gig as the spokesperson for the company that makes the stuff! Just one more example of how being honest pays off.

**Simon Cowell** has been quoted saying, "Yes, I've had Botox [Cosmetic], but not in an obsessive way. Then again, every guy I know who works in the City [London] has had it now." I love it when men 'fess up to cosmetic intervention.

What's next for Simon? How about a breast reduction?

## ( Three )

# Plump It Up: Lips

Joan woke up having dreamt she was Angelina Jolie with luscious, bee-stung lips, a back tattoo, a variety of cute adopted children, and a permanent pillow next to Brad Pitt. She knew realistically her lips would have to be the first thing she tried to achieve on her wish list in order to look better. But sadly, one look in the mirror confirmed that her own lips were thinner than the Earth's ozone layer. Joan was determined, however, to get a big fat pucker without cosmetic or surgical enhancement.

Since she wasn't personally acquainted with any beekeepers, she went straight to the grocery store and launched Plan B. Nestled between the kumquats and Minneola tangelos, Joan proceeded to suck the juice out of every lemon in the produce section, hoping her lips would plump up and men would line up from as far away as aisle seven to kiss them.

It didn't happen, and Joan came to the conclusion quickly that the only way to make lemonade out of her lemon lips was going to be with the help *of a dermatologist (plus the money from her mother's bosom). The next day she went in for her very first lip injections.*

Pink, soft, smooth, plump, and juicy.

Do I have your attention?

I'm not talking about strawberries. I'm talking about lips. The pair on your face. The kissers. Men are transfixed by sexy lips. If he could, a man would stare at a woman's luscious lips all day long, with only short breaks to divert his attention to her boobs. If you have succulent, tantalizing lips, a man will gladly watch you talk for hours on a first date, without falling asleep in his pasta.

By the way, no matter how sexy your lips are, a first date is not the best time to tell a man about your deep-seated fear of snakes. Or hot dogs. Or cigars. Or garden hoses. Or anything tubular.

Save that for your wedding night.

And we all know why men love to gaze longingly at a woman's mouth. If you can't imagine why, read my lips: Vagina!

That's why most women try never to go without makeup on their lips. It's also why some men like women with mustaches. The lips on your face give him something to fantasize about as a substitute for other ones. You can't very well enjoy a dinner date while standing on your head, naked from the waist down (or should I say "up"?).

However, in a highly unscientific study I conducted among the straight men I know, 90 percent of them admitted that if they could, they'd be thrilled to engage in dinner conversation with their wives' and girlfriends' vulvas, as a refreshing change.

The ancient Egyptians were aware of the upper lips/lower lips connection. They created the world's first version of lipstick and painted their mouths to look red and succulent, to resemble other parts. Cleopatra's own blend of lip enhancement was a deep-red mash of crushed beetles and ants.

Her lips were crawling with color.

And, as history confirms, the leaders of the Roman Empire, Julius

Caesar and Mark Antony, men who could have had any woman—including those with smaller, more feminine noses—chose Cleopatra and her bugged-out lips.

Modern-day Cleo wannabes, the models and actresses who appear in ads, movies, and TV shows, are constantly photographed sucking lollipops, eating strawberries and bananas. A lot of candy and fruit looks phallic. It's Seduction 101. A woman with sexy lips can put *anything* in her mouth, and men swoon with desire.

Men are dumbstruck by the sight of beautiful lips. We all know the legend of Cupid, the son of Aphrodite, who would shoot an arrow with his bow into the heart of a man, making him fall madly in love with the first woman he saw. Here's what you might not know: The top lip, with its double-arch shape, is called "Cupid's bow." Beautiful lips are a woman's love-striking weapon. Smile and pierce the heart.

Your lips can say "sexy" without moving. They can say "tomato" and still be saying "sexy." Not that a man is actually listening to the words. He's staring at your pucker. Having fully articulated lips not only makes you attractive to men, it makes the woman feel sexy, too. Even Grandma knew it. That's why she always said, "Go put on some lipstick, honey. You'll feel better."

One of the added benefits of having big beautiful lips is that they're a constant reminder of how good you look. You feel their plumpness wrapped around every word. You wouldn't be able to forget them if you tried. And all that mental focus on one body part—how good they look, how soft they feel, how nice it'd be to use them—can be a huge turn-on for you, too.

When you look in the mirror, do you feel that your lips are on the thin side? Are they kissers that lack enough cushion to absorb a juicy smooch from the man you love or admire? All of our features send subconscious messages to the world, and lips are important communicators—even if we don't say a word. Thin lips on a woman give the wrong impression, of shrewishness and prudishness, and probably other "ishnesses" that are the opposite of alluring and desirable.

It's unfair to be thought of as frigid or sexless just because you have thin lips. Your lips have just as many nerve endings as Angelina "Pelican Mouth" Jolie's. Kissing feels as good to you as it does to Paris "Trout Pout" Hilton.

Regardless, when a man sees swollen lips, he believes the owner is sexual and passionate.

And useful, too! In a car crash, you've got built-in air bags on your face.

The chubbiness of lips is determined by both your genes and your age. Either you have a thin-lipped legacy, or you suffer from age-related loss of lip volume.* As we get older, a lot of areas in the face lose their cushy fat pads of youth: the cheeks, the space under the eye—and the lips. It's a process called lipoatrophy.

Now here's a sad fact: People, as they age, actually lose weight in their lips! The one place you want more of it. Other factors that thin lips over time are:

1. Sun exposure saps the collagen and elastin fibers that make lips firm and pliant. Go find an SPF 344 sunblock lipstick today!
2. Smoking! Every time you put a cigarette to your lips, the smoke and sucking movement carve lines around your mouth, and saps the springiness out of your skin.

Therefore, if you *wanted* to prematurely age your lips, smoking cigarettes in the sun is the fastest way to do it.

To plump up lips, you've got several options. None of them is hard to handle, as you'll see below. Whichever option you consider, they're all good for feeling sexier, more confident, and eager to get more mileage out of your mouth.

*By the time Angelina Jolie is ninety, she'll weigh only ten pounds.

# Lip Implants

**What are they made of and how do they work?** A biocompatible substance (meaning that it will be accepted by your body without a fight) is inserted into your lips to add volume. There are a few ways to do this.

The first is the synthetic implant category. We have **Gore-Tex®** (yes, it *is* the same stuff your ski parka is made of) and **SoftForm,** both of which are porous versions of Teflon. Their Swiss-cheese structure allows the right kind of scar tissue to form in the holes, holding the implant in place, but not deforming the shape of your lips.

The second is the natural category. We have **AlloDerm®**, purified collagen made from human cadavers (all screened exhaustively for diseases). The collagen is rolled into a sheet and shaped according to need. It can be—and is—used on any body part, including gums in dental surgery, and it's the implant of choice for phalloplasty, more commonly known as penis enlargement surgery.

And though it may not be appropriate here, I always think that when her Alloderm lips meet his Alloderm penis, it's like a family reunion.

Last, the recently FDA-approved **Artefill®** is both part implant and part filler. Artefill is made of microscopic plastic beads suspended in purified cow collagen. Once injected into the lips, the cow collagen is slowly absorbed by the body, while the micro-beads stimulate natural collagen to form around them.

Here's the 411 on synthetic and natural lip implants:

**How does the implant get in there?** The doctor injects the implant into the corner of the lips with a needle and then shapes the material with his fingers. The procedure is quick. Less than an hour. A local anesthetic that numbs the lips is given before the implant goes in, so it's relatively painless as it's being done.

**Does it last?** Implants, like diamonds and pre-nups, are forever.

**Pain?** Any pain, swelling, and discomfort should be gone within a week.

**Drawbacks?** Every procedure has risks. The risks of lip implants are lumps, numbness, an asymmetrical pout, infection (the implant might have to come out), and/or migration (the implant will have to be repositioned).

**Benefits?** Implants are not going to leave you one day for a younger mouth. It's a one-time expense.

**$$$?** It'll cost between $2,000 and $5,000.

**What if I hate it?** No worries! Implants are made of material that is as easy to remove as it is to put in. Should you decide that the implants make you look like you've been sucking on a vacuum, or that so much new attention from men is a terrible burden, then make an appointment with your doctor. He'll get them out without too much hassle.

**Aftercare?** There is none, so relax and go lipstick shopping. Implants are permanent. You won't need to do anything but lap up the attention and kiss as many men as possible until you're too pooped to pucker.

## Fat Transfer for the Lips

**What is it?** Fat is removed from a place you don't need it (butt, hips, belly, thighs), and injected into the lips.

**How's it done?** Robert Singer, M.D., veteran plastic surgeon of San Diego, explained it to me: "I start by taking available fat from the buttock, hip, or belly with a syringe or a small cannula," he said. "For the lips, only a small amount is needed—five ccs per lip—but I take about four times more because the fat has a lot of fluid. Before injecting the fat into the lips, doctors treat it first. Some wash it with saline to get rid of any liquefied fat, broken cells, and impurities. Some doctors put the fat in a centrifuge to separate it into three layers. On top, it's liquefied fat. On the bottom, it's saline. In the middle are usable dense fat cells. The doctor puts them in a needle and injects pinpoint amounts into the lip at different places in multiple layers.

"There's an artistry to it. You don't want to inject a glob or get too much volume," he said. Of all the fat injected, 30 to 50 percent will stick. The rest is absorbed by the body. Your lips will look progressively smaller, until they level off. Because of shrinkage, your doctor will overfill at first.

**Does it last?** Fat transfers are considered semi-permanent.* Fat cells that survive the transfer hook up with vessels to create a blood supply and aren't going anywhere in a hurry—years, if ever.

**Pain?** Minilipo of the butt? Then lots of needle pricks in the lips? Yeah, it hurts, but you'll get local numbing.

**Drawbacks?** The big problem with fat transfer is the unpredictability of it. You might be one of those people to get adequate fat shots into your lips, but at least thirty percent of it just won't take. It'll be absorbed back into the body, and your lips won't look significantly different than before.

**Benefits?** There's a nice organic aspect to fat transfer. I like the idea of using your own material, recycling your own fat.

Al Gore would approve.

Plus, there is no chance of your body having an allergic reaction or rejecting its own cells. It's just a question of whether they can tolerate the move.

**$$$$?** A bit pricey because it's a multi-step process, with local anesthesia in two places. Expect a bill of $3,000 to $5,000. Also, if the fat doesn't take, you'll either have to do it again (and pay again), or try something else (which won't be free either).

**What if I hate it?** Since you'll be over-stuffed, assuming that at least a third of the fat will be absorbed, your lips will feel too full for a short time. Give it a week; let nature take its course. On the off chance that you are the one person in the world who retains *all* of

---

*like most Hollywood marriages

your transferred fat, you can always have lip liposuction to take it down a notch.

**Aftercare?** Smile with your new, full mouth. In six months or so, according to Dr. Singer, you'll have lost some of the weight, and might want a booster transfer.

# Fillers for Lips

**What are they?** Fillers are natural or synthetic injectable substances that will plump your lips for up to six months.

We'll start with your basic **human-derived collagen.** Collagen is a protein that is already in our skin, giving it firmness. By injecting a manufactured needleful of it into your lips, it's just putting back what the sun, smoking, and age have taken away. Brand names include **Cosmoderm®** and **Cosmoplast™**.

**Bovine-derived collagen** is a collagen that comes from cows. Unlike the human-derived type, you might have an allergic reaction to the cow collagen, and it should be tested before it's shot into your lips. Brand names include **Zyderm®** and **Zyplast®**.

Last, we have **hyaluronic acid fillers.** Hyaluronic acid, like collagen, is produced by your body, but as we age, we produce less. This molecule is a sponge-like carbohydrate that naturally binds to water. So, when a hyaluronic acid filler is injected under your skin, the area inflates with fluid. It's like retaining water, but just on the lips. Have no fear. You won't slosh when you talk, but you will have fuller lips, with a well-defined Cupid's bow, aka the double-curved upper lip. Two popular brand names are **Restylane®** and **Juvéderm™ Ultra.**

Here are the basics on lip fillers:

**How's it done?** Depending on the filler you and your doctor choose, you might get a numbing shot or a topical anesthetic. I can say from personal experience, collagen injections hurt. By all means, ask for an anesthetic!

Then the doctor injects the filler at strategic points for uniform plumping. He'll massage a bit, to distribute the filler. Then you'll be cleaned at the injection sites. And that's it. Be warned: Doctors have to overfill lips with collagen because a lot of it dissipates. When I do it, my lips look amazing for a week. After that, they look better, but not as full. From start to finish, the procedure takes less than half an hour.

**Does it last?** Collagen, sadly, only turns up the lip volume for several months. Hyaluronic acid fillers can last longer, but don't hold your breath (even with those puffy lips) for them to last beyond six months.

**Pain?** Collagen injections usually contain lidocaine, a painkilling agent. Even with that, as I've said, try to get extra numbing! You'll be glad you did. Hyaluronic acid fillers don't have painkiller mixed in. You'll want something for numbing before the injections of Restylane and Hylaform.

**Drawbacks?** With the cow products, you'll need allergy testing a month before the injections. With any filler, you'll have some redness, swelling, and maybe bruising, itching, and tenderness.

**Benefits?** Perhaps the words "inexpensive" and "easy" ring a bell for you? Also, how about "instant" and "sexy"?

**$$?** Collagen fillers will run you about $500 per syringe. Hyaluronic acid fillers shots are $600 a syringe.

**What if I hate it?** Wait several months.

**Aftercare?** Schedule your lip job appointments twice a year. Or, if you really, *really* love it, think about the long term. Spending $600 every six months for Restylane might not be as cost-effective as dropping $5,000 *once* for implants. A lot of women use fillers to sample a taste of red-hot juicy lips. Before long, a taste isn't enough, and they upgrade to implants.

# Celeb Lip Ticker

## In the Bee-Stung category:

**Lindsay Lohan:** She's a messed-up kid, but she's got gorgeous lips.

**Keira Knightley:** Painfully thin, everywhere, except her luscious mouth.

**Courteney Cox:** Gets better-looking as she ages by adding volume where she needs it; in this case, her lips.

## In the Swarm-Attack category:

**Dyan Cannon:** Living proof that big lips should stop at fifty. Cannon is too old for an inner-tube mouth. Now she looks like a Chinese frog. You want to put a coin between her lips.

**Lisa Rinna:** She's making a career now out of being a Cougar, with the plumped-up lips to rival younger women.

**Angelina Jolie:** Poster girl for exploding lips. In the final scenes of *Girl, Interrupted,* her lips looked painful! I recently saw her on the red carpet, and her lips were as big as a pelican's. I wanted to throw fish at her.

**Paris Hilton:** Maybe her huge mouth will distract people from all of the stupid things that come out of it.*

**Meg Ryan:** There was adorable Meg before lip implants and desperate Meg after. The bigger her lips, the smaller her box office. Too much of a good thing? Yup.

**Jenna Jameson:** With lips like that, who needs air bags?

*And go into it.

# Four

# Filler Up: Wrinkles

*Joan wasn't getting any younger, and she had the wrinkles to prove it. Though Botox had helped to smooth the fine lines on her forehead and around her mouth, the doctor insisted it was a bad idea to inject her with Botox Cosmetics around the eyes (it could leave her with that terrible partial stroke, Mary Jo Buttafuoco look). This was horrible, as the crow's feet around her eyes were so big they had varicose veins. So she was thrilled to learn that dermal fillers injected into the skin would eliminate them. But again, that meant injections, and Joan hated needles!*

*Joan decided she was going to do it her way, so she went to the Home Depot for some caulking. She figured if it could keep a shower in a pre-war walk up from leaking and looking brand new, surely it could smooth out her rough edges.*

*Once inside the Home Depot, with the help of a butch lesbian couple shopping for lumber for their new shed, she was directed to what she needed for her own secret fountain of youth: acrylic bathtub caulk! Joan had a choice to make, though: beige or fawn? She selected the sealant that most resembled her complexion and generously applied it to the avian footprints around her eyes. The caulk was nice and dry when she arrived home. Joan excitedly wiped the caulk from her crow's feet only to be struck with horror to see that the result resembled the dirty grout of a crackhouse bathroom. She knew it was time to call a dermatologist, and quickly!!*

Clear, smooth skin is the foundation of beauty. We call makeup "foundation" for this reason. A shining, radiant face—unlined and well rounded—triggers just about every receptor in a man's reptilian brain. When he sees a fresh-faced woman, he instantly knows she's well fed, healthy, active, young, fertile, carefree, and not tormented by crushing anxieties. (Men are pre-programmed to avoid women with "issues.") An open face is an open invitation.

Our skin is our canvas. Even perfect facial features don't look good on spotty, wrinkled, and sagging skin. You could have the biggest, juiciest lips in creation, but they wouldn't look so alluring if rimmed with cracks and tiny creases. The most adorable nose in the world doesn't look so delicate with deep trenches extending down from the nostrils to the corners of your mouth. Your forehead might be ivory, but it won't gleam in the light with gash-like horizontal wrinkles running across it.

Fine lines are not fine at all. Okay, yes, yes, I've heard the argument for lines and wrinkles, that they're "badges of honor," the "sign that you've lived a rich, full life," or that you "demonstrate your feelings with your face." Congrats for being an emotional person. But most of that was said *before* facial fillers arrived on the scene.

Now, we no longer need to justify the existence of wrinkles . . . we can get rid of them!

Although emotions and expressions are how we experience our lives and communicate with others, they wreak havoc on your skin. Make an expression enough times, it'll be etched on your face. The parentheses between your eyebrows? Frown lines. Smile a lot? You'll get crow's feet, the lines by the corner of your eyes that look like bird footprints in wet cement.*

Some of you might remember an old "Twilight Zone" episode, one of my faves, where relatives of a dying man were told they'd get their hands on his fortune only if they spent the entire night in his mansion wearing hideous masks. The masks were exaggerated versions of their true personalities: pathetic, morose, hateful, angry. Anyway, the greedy relatives all stuck it out in the mansion until morning and were granted their inheritance. But when they took off the masks? Their faces had turned into the masks' shapes. They were rich but doomed by horrible, disfigured faces.

This show was made, clearly, in the days before plastic surgery. Nowadays, the greedy relatives could wear the masks, take the money, and then spend a chunk of it fixing their faces back.

I tell this story because, by age sixty, our faces *do* turn into the masks of our true personality.

I've never tried the popular filler Restylane. It lasts a long time, but you get bruising, so that doesn't work for me. I do collagen injections, however: I can get a shot in the morning, and I can be on camera in the afternoon. I also have some collagen on my chin to get rid of dimples. It's not a Shirley Temple dimple. More Shirley Bassey. Also, I've had injections around my lips.

It's a tragedy to have smoker's lips when you don't even smoke. . . like doing the time without committing the crime.

Our faces are maps of our expressions. Luckily these days, for many women, that map leads them directly to a good dermatologist, who has fillers to erase the lines, take a decade off their faces, and recalibrate the way the world looks at them and—most importantly—how they look at themselves.

All this can be yours for less than a thousand dollars. Go ahead and smile. Those crow's feet can't hurt you anymore.

---

*My own crow's feet were so bad they had bunions.

# Where Do Wrinkles Come From?

From HELL, of course.

Besides habitual facial muscle action, there are four main skin enemies: 1) sun damage, 2) smoking, 3) gravity, and 4) aging.

1. Sun damage. You know how putting a plant under a sun light makes it grow faster? Well, spending a lot of time in the sun does the same thing to your face, making it *age* faster.

   Therefore, the only times it's safe to leave your house are after dark and/or during a solar eclipse.

   The UVA and UVB rays are especially damaging when you're young, before age twenty. That wicked sunburn from Daytona, Spring Break '85 can't be undone. Sun damage after age twenty? It's not as severe, but be careful just the same. Besides causing wrinkles, the sun also causes cancer.

   Who cares if you've got gorgeously tanned skin if you're dead? But if you're still alive, use an SPF 15 moisturizer . . . every day! You can't be too careful. If I could, I'd use SPF 322,000. (In a confusing twist, now doctors are telling women to get more Vitamin D and are recommending they sit in sunlight for fifteen to twenty minutes a day! Consider it the RDA of daytime.)

2. Smoking. What's even worse than lying out on the beach? Doing it with a cigarette in your mouth. Can I just say, not to lecture, that smoking is like committing harakiri to your skin. You might as well stick the lit end of the cigarette into your cheek. A decade of smoking will do no worse. The smoke literally draws out precious moisture and stymies collagen production, drying your skin and sapping its strength, especially around the mouth.

What man is going to want to kiss a pair of cracked, withered, grandma lips—when you're only thirty-five?

For your skin's sake, quit smoking. Otherwise, don't blame me when, for your lips, forty is the new eighty.

3. Gravity. Well, it's no rainbow. Your face droops and sags, just like your boobs and behind. The natural pull toward the center of the earth would not be so bad if your skin weren't progressively weaker, too. Which brings me to . . .

4. Aging. As we get older, our production of collagen (what makes your skin firm) and elastin (what makes it springy) slows down. Without as much connective tissue holding our skin up, fighting gravity is next to impossible. Your skin can only take so much of the onslaught before it succumbs.

And that, dear reader, is where wrinkles come from.

How to send them *back* to hell? Read on.

## Cracks, Crevices, and Canyons

Each wrinkle is unique. They're like orgasms. Some are deep. Some are shallow. Others make you scream. Unlike orgasms, however, when even a bad one is still pretty good, there's no such thing as a good wrinkle. They're all bad, unless you're a shar-pei.

Wrinkles come in a variety of styles:

1. The least horrible are called **lines**. They're shallow and thin, little whispers that say, "I'm barely noticeable *now*, but just you wait!"

2. The basics are called **wrinkles**, deeper and clearly visible on your forehead, around the eyes and lips.

3.  The biggest kind are called **folds**. There are the deepest creases, including the nasolabial fold, which is the trench that runs from your nose to the corners of your mouth.

Another set of folds is charmingly referred to as "marionette" or "Howdy Doody" lines, which extend from the corners of your mouth down to your chin. They make you look like a wooden puppet with a moveable mouth that's saying, "Help me! Help me!"

The easiest way to identify the distinction between lines, wrinkles, and folds is their depth . . . as in, how deeply you hate them.

A quickie reminder from medical school: Our skin, the six-pound organ of human tissue that covers our entire body, has many purposes. Protection, insulation, regulating temperature, providing a home for hair follicles and sweat glands. It comprises three main layers: the epidermis is what we show or hide from the world, our birthday suit; the middle part, or dermis, is connective tissue, the infrastructure of our skin; underneath the dermis is a subcutaneous layer of fat that cushions our skin against the muscle beneath that.

Aging (and for sun goddesses and smokers, make that *premature* aging) takes place on all three skin levels. It's a systematic breakdown. On top, the epidermis loses 10 percent of its cells per decade. Fewer cells mean the skin gets thinner. The thinner the skin, the less it's able to hold moisture.

No moisture = dryness.

Dryness = wrinkles.

Got it?

In the middle, the dermal layer takes a staggering hit by the passage of time. The dermis's collagen and elastin fibers, the network of support that holds your skin together, gets thin and stretched. Imagine a once-taut circus net slowly sagging and sinking to the sawdust-sprinkled floor. Also, sweat glands' productivity slows, and your natural oil reserves dry up.

I don't need to repeat—but I will—that dryness is next to wrinkliness.

Last, the fat layer underneath your skin also thins with age. Ordinarily, I'd say, "Great." Thin is in. But, on your face, the fat layer fills out wrinkles and holds up your cheeks, forehead, and chin. Without fat to fill you out, wrinkles will show in high relief, and your skin will sag, which creates not only *more* wrinkles, but deep, devastating folds.

As a veteran of the anti-aging war, it's my duty to deliver the harsh truth about skin aging. I don't like doing it. But I feel I must. Nature has a way of robbing us of our youth, bit by bit, and that's the sad reality of life.

Fortunately, the happy reality of science is that we can turn back the clock with a needle.

## Get Your Filler

Dermal fillers are the rage. Why? They do for you what over-the-counter creams and lotions *wish* they could, but don't. The use of injectable fillers is often called a "liquid face lift." You can take five to ten years off your face, for a fraction of the cost of surgery, with hardly any risk. No knives. Only needles.

That said, fillers are great for forty-five-year-old women who want to look thirty-five. Not so great for sixty-five-year-old women who want to look fifty-five. By the time you're sixty, using fillers won't be enough. You can't rebuild an entire house using caulk. You need beams, bricks, the heavy-duty structural goods that a surgical face lift can provide. (See Chapter 7: About Face Lifts).

We all know what happens when a trend gets popular. The marketplace is *flooded* with product. Everyone—and his grandmother, her dog, and the dog's grandmother—wants a piece of the action. In the twenty years since collagen was first injected into a woman's face, dozens of facial fillers have become available. And dozens more are on the way. What I'm including in the filler round-up that follows are the tried and true, time-tested, people-friendly fillers that I, or friends of mine, have personally used with good results. You'll notice that some of these fillers were mentioned in the previous chapter on lip augmentation. The ones listed here are for wrinkles and folds, not necessarily lips.

"Since there are so many fillers out there, it does seem hard to choose which one to use," said my friend, Michigan-based surgeon Anthony Youn, M.D., author of the highly entertaining blog Celebrity Cosmetic Surgery. "Fortunately, your doctor knows each one, what it's best for, and can recommend one based on his preferences and experiences. Other factors to take into account are how long you want the filler to last, how much pain you can handle, how much recovery time you have, what type of wrinkles need to be filled. There are so many variables, and once you address each one, a filler will emerge as the best choice for the situation."

I've made a pretty comprehensive list. Your doctor might be in love with something I haven't included.* Fine. If you trust him—and you will, having screened him carefully—then listen to his pitch and research the product on your own. Should it check out, go for it! All told, almost 1.5 million people had soft-tissue fillers in 2007. And, as far as I know, they're all smiling.

**One warning flag about fillers:** Use products that are legal in the United States. A product that's injected into the face of five million Frenchwomen might be *fantastique*—in France. But this ain't France. It's the good old U.S.A., so stick with the FDA-approved list.

*like his secretary

## Category One: Human Collagen

**Cosmoderm/Cosmoplast:** It's practically the same stuff that's been in your skin your whole life, except it's purified and grows in a laboratory. Use human collagen products for any line, wrinkle, or fold on the face, including frown lines, crow's feet, forehead lines, marionette lines, lip cracks, and nasolabial folds. For the deep etch marks, use Cosmoplast. For lighter ironing, go with Cosmoderm.

**Rx:** No pre-allergy test required. After the doctor cleans the area, he'll inject the syringe into the wrinkle or fold, massage the area for equal distribution, and that's it. Collagen usually comes with lidocaine mixed in, but, like I always say, if you're wimpy about pain (like me!), get extra local anesthesia along with it.

There are side effects like redness, swelling, bruising, maybe some small lumps, but they'll fade. In fact, about half of the collagen injected fades after the first few days. You'll be over-inflated at the doc's office, and then settle down in the days to come.

**$$:** Around $500 per syringe. Depending on how many areas you want treated, you might need two syringes. In terms of annual cost, you'll have to reinject every three or four months. So call it, on the low end, $2,000 a year.

**Dr. Youn's Expert Opinion:** "With longer-lasting options out there, collagen is largely obsolete. I don't use it in my practice anymore. But it does have the advantage of a quick recovery time. It's for 'right now,' to look good tonight."

## Category Two: Bovine Collagen

**Zyplast/Zyderm:** These were the first collagen products to receive FDA approval for treatment of wrinkles anywhere on the face and lips. Both are made from bovine collagen. That means cow. You're not injecting a porterhouse steak into your crow's feet, but rather the dermal fiber that once sat atop a juicy, raw porterhouse. Hope that eases your mind.

**Word of warning:** Don't try this in India where cows are considered holy.

**Rx:** A month before injection, you should be tested for an allergic reaction. It's cow, after all. Some people's bodies don't appreciate the bovine invasion. If you have no reaction, the doctor will inject the syringe into the wrinkle or fold, massage the area for equal distribution, and that's it. You'll look udderly fabulous. As with human-derived collagen, the side effects include redness, swelling, and bruising.* About half of it fades after the first few days.

**$$:** Like its human equivalent, the results last only three or four months. For a year's worth of wrinkle plumping, at $500/syringe a quarter, expect to pay a baseline of $2,000.

**Dr. Youn's Expert Opinion:** "Same as human-derived collagen. It doesn't last as long as other options, and it's just as expensive. Plus, you have to wait a month to clear the allergy test. But it's reliable, safe, and effective, with a fast recovery time."

**Hot off the presses!** In the near future, look for the product **Evolence,** an FDA-approval-pending porcine collagen product.

Warning: Though you'll squeal with delight, it might make your face smell like bacon.

## Category Three: Hyaluronic Acid

Hyaluronic acid is a carbohydrate that we produce naturally in our bodies. Its main job is to act as a sponge, absorbing a thousand times its weight in water. The problem of dehydration? Fixed. Problem of dryness? Nixed. Hyaluronic acid also latches onto collagen and elastin, giving those fibers nutrients and liquid to make them play at the top of their game. There are many of these types of filler out there.

---

*and in the odd instance, an uncontrollable desire to moo

**Preville Silk** and **Captique**™: Two brand-new options in the hyaluronic-filler class. Preville Silk is the first one to have lidocaine built in, to ease pain in injection. Early reports are that Preville goes in as thin and smooth as silk (hence the name), and is virtually painless with no recovery time. Same with Captique. Easy in, then go out. Both are plant-based, or non-animal-derived, so you won't need pretesting for allergies.

**Rx:** The advantage is such ease in injection—no numbing needed, just insert, squirt, and put on your dancing dress—and no recovery. You'll be good to go as soon as the needle's removed, without swelling, bruising, or redness.

**$:** Only $400 to $500 a syringe sounds reasonable. But since these two last up to ninety days, you'll be visiting the doctor's office and the ATM frequently.

**Dr. Youn's Expert Opinion:** "They're both marketed as 'today for tonight' fillers. I think of them as the lighter category of filler. They're thinner, easy to inject, less painful, less trauma when injected, no recovery time, but they last only three months. You get these and look good right away. I wouldn't use them on deep folds and wrinkles, though."

**Restylane:** As close to a gold standard as there is in facial fillers, Restylane is a non-animal-derived hyaluronic acid. In other words, it's made in a lab using ingredients not found on any creature with a face. Vegans can use it with a clear conscience. This stuff is great for the lips, mouth wrinkles, adding volume to the eye areas, the brows, the cheeks, plumping up wrinkles and folds. Doctors are now using it to add volume to noses, soften old-looking hands, and even in the area under the eyes to disguise dark circles.

**Rx:** No allergy testing needed, but you will appreciate some local numbing at the injection site first. The doctor injects directly into the wrinkle or near it and then massages the area for equal distribution. Expect redness, bruising, swelling, a bit of pain and tenderness for a day or two. Worst-case scenario: The doctor injected too close to the surface of your skin, you can see and feel the filler.

**$$:** A bit pricier than collagen, at $600/syringe. You'll go back for more every six months, to the tune of $1,200 a year minimum.

**Dr. Youn's Expert Opinion:** "I use a lot of Restylane in my practice. The advantages are that it lasts longer than collagen, doesn't fade after a few days, and you can use it anywhere, on all wrinkle types. The disadvantages are that it's more expensive, hurts more, and has a longer recovery time. Basically, the longer a filler lasts, the bigger the needle, the more it hurts when injected, and the greater the reaction risks. Restylane is a jack-of-all-trades middle-category filler."

**Juvéderm Ultra:** The first hyaluronic acid filler to win FDA approval all the way back in 2001, Juvéderm Ultra, which is a gel, is a time-tested winner. Use it to treat all facial wrinkles and folds, around the mouth, eyes, forehead, chin, what have you. Juvéderm can also add volume where needed: under the eyes, to raise scars, to round off hollowed cheeks. Juvéderm Ultra Plus is the same stuff, with bigger particles for deeper wrinkles.

**Rx:** No allergy testing needed. You will want some local numbing shots or a topical numbing application before injecting. The doctor injects, massages, and then you walk out the door. Expect redness, bruising, swelling, possible tenderness, itching, and pain for a few days. Worst-case scenario: if a hasty doctor inserts the needle too close to the surface of your skin, you might be able to see and feel the filler, or small bumps under the skin.

**$$:** About $600 per syringe. It'll last for six months and cost $1,200 per year, at least.

**Dr. Youn's Expert Opinion:** "I put Juvéderm Ultra in the same category as Restylane. If there is any difference between the two, Juvéderm Ultra is a little softer. I use Juvéderm Ultra for anything, shallow or deep wrinkles."

**Perlane®** and **Juvéderm Ultra Plus:** These two have thicker gel particles than the other hyaluronic fillers, making them like Restylane and Juvéderm Ultra on steroids. Its bigger particles work better on deeper wrinkles and folds. They're used for all the same problems as the middle-category fillers—wrinkles, folds, to increase volume where needed—but for more severe cases.

**Rx:** No allergy testing needed, but, believe me, you will appreciate local numbing at the injection site first. Same drill you've heard already. The doctor injects directly into the wrinkle, or near it, and massages for equal distribution. You'll have the same recovery risks, but amplified, and longer-lasting. Expect redness, bruising, swelling, a bit of pain and tenderness for a week. Worst-case scenario: The doctor injected too close to the surface of your skin, you can see or feel the filler; a particular worry, considering Perlane and Juvéderm Ultra Plus's thicknesses.

**$$:** Only slightly more expensive than Restylane, at $650 per syringe, but the results last twice as long.

**Dr. Youn's Expert Opinion:** "I put these in the heavy category, which means more expensive, more pain, bigger needle, longer recovery. Perlane has bigger particles, so it's grittier. You can't use it on shallow wrinkles, and you do have a higher risk of lumps. For deep wrinkles, though, these both work well, and last a long, long time."

## Category Four: Synthetic Microspheres

**Artefill®** mixes two concepts to create one giant step forward for womankind. It's made of tiny polymethylmethacrylate microspheres (a synthetic polymer used in surgical implants), suspended in bovine collagen. Think of it like a peanut M&M. The peanut center is the implant material that lasts forever, and the crunchy bovine collagen coating stimulates the growth of your own collagen. The results are permanent. Or, in other words, "non-reabsorbable."

**Rx:** Cow allergy testing is needed beforehand. Once you clear that hurdle, you're ready to proceed. After some cleaning of the facial areas, your doctor will inject Artefill into the site. It already has lidocaine built in, but you might want extra painkiller. The doctor might be conservative with the amount because it's permanent. Better to add more later than worry about putting too much in. You'll walk out a bit swollen and bruised. The wrinkles look improved immediately, and they'll continue to improve over the next six months as your own new collagen has had a chance to grow.

**$$$:** Higher, but cost-effective. An Artefill treatment might run you up to $2,000. But it's a one time expense. One Artefill injection costs less than two years of hyaluronic filler shots.

**Dr. Youn's Expert Opinion:** "Permanent does sound good, I know. But a lot of doctors aren't fond of permanent. If you inject it in the wrong place, or the patient doesn't like it, the only option is to cut it out. Also, when people age, their faces change. The filler might look good at fifty, but at sixty, it's not in the right place and looks strange. There's always the risk of infection, even five years down the road. And the last disadvantage to Artefill is the allergy testing period. You have a couple of months to wait before a doctor can inject."

## Category Five: Calcium Hydroxylapatite

**Radiesse®** is made from calcium-based microspheres, a substance found in bones and teeth, suspended in a water-based gel. Like Artefill, Radiesse stimulates the growth of your own collagen, so the results continue to improve and last a lot longer than collagen and hyaluronic acid fillers. It's great for all wrinkles and folds, but keep it away from the lips! It tends to get lumpy there.

**Rx:** No allergy tests. No numbing agent needed. You'll be cleaned, and injected with Radiesse. You hear "calcium" and you might think "calcify." Have no fear. The stuff stays soft. It won't go hard in you. In fact, it takes on the texture of the surrounding tissue, like the Predator in the Arnold Schwarzenegger movie. Basically, it blends and lasts for a year or more.

**$$$:** Pricey. Up to $1,500 a syringe. But, as it's good for a year, it works out to be roughly the same price as a hyaluronic acid filler.

**Dr. Youn's Expert Opinion:** "It's basically a bone paste. I don't use it. I think Perlane is close enough to the same results. Not to slam Radiesse. I'm just more comfortable with Perlane. Another doctor might be more comfortable with Radiesse. It's a personal preference. Coke or Pepsi."

## Category Six: Synthetic Poly-L-Lactic Acid

Sculptra™ was originally intended to treat lipoatrophy (facial fat loss) for HIV patients. Now it's being used to plump up the cheeks in perfectly healthy people. And why not? It works like a dream on wrinkles and folds, too. It's made of millions of microspheres of the same chemical used in dissolving surgical sutures. We produce poly-L-lactic acid in our bodies naturally. The synthetic variety is biocompatible (meaning it gets along great with human tissue). When it's injected, it thickens skin and fluffs up sad, depressed areas, like hollows and wrinkles.

**Rx:** No allergy testing is needed here, but you'll want that hit of lidocaine before you get multiple shots around the treatment areas. There's a bit of bruising, redness, and swelling. Next step, do it again five more times, every six weeks. But after that, you're good for two years. The results come on you gradually, as you produce your own collagen, and as more and more of the poly-L-lactic acid is injected.

**$$$$:** Another pricey one. A hit of Sculptra costs $600, and you need multiple syringes at each of your six sessions to see the best results. Calculators out: That's $3,600 *minimum*.

**Dr. Youn's Expert Opinion:** "Sculptra is really only for revolumizing the face, to fill out hollow areas. It's not really practical to fill wrinkles. You can use Sculptra on deep folds, but it won't be as effective as Restylane, and it's a lot more expensive."

## Category Seven: Fat (your own)

If you want to add fat to your face, you might as well use some of what you've got on your butt. I mean, it's already there, and would be honored to make better use of itself than being sat on.

A **fat transfer** is when you take fat from one place (that can spare it, like the butt, thighs, or belly), and put it in your cheeks, or lips, or wrinkles, or eye hollows. No way will you have an allergic reaction to the fat that's been thriving on your belly for twenty years. Like a plant that grows beautifully in one space, however, it might not like being moved to another spot. The transferred fat needs to find a blood supply in its new home, or it'll die and be absorbed by the body. It's a dramatic race against time, actually. The cells will live three or four days without blood. And it takes three or four days for the transplanted fat to hook up with a new supplier. About half of it won't survive the trip. The half that does? It sticks for a year or more.

**Rx:** The first step is for the doctor to take fat from where you don't need it—butt, belly, hips, your call. Then he'll purify the fat to get good, dense fat cells to transfer. Next, he'll put the good cells in a syringe, and make a series of pinpoint injections into your wrinkles in multiple layers. Of all the fat injected, 30 to 50 percent will stick. The rest is absorbed by the body. Typically, a doctor purposefully adds too much fat, expecting much of it to die. You'll have to wait four days to see what your wrinkles or lips are going to look like from now on.

**$$$$:** The fat transfer is a multi-step, multi-tool, double dose of painkiller, two-stage production here. Which means? You pay more for it. A lot more. Up to $5,000. But it's semi-permanent. Some of the fat will hang around forever. But over time, most of it will eventually be absorbed by the body. It's all organic. Recycling your own fat for better use? Al Gore would be thrilled.

**Dr. Youn's Expert Opinion:** "Fat grafting is better for filling in facial hollows, to revolumize sunken areas. For wrinkles and folds, it's a lot less expensive and easier to use than a filler like Restylane."

Less expensive and easy? That's speaking my language.

## Holy Moles

I can't stand moles. I know the eighteenth-century French found them sexy.* Not me. When I see a mole on someone's face, I just want to swat it.

I've never understood why the signature mole is so sexy. But I might be alone there. Marilyn Monroe had one. Would Cindy Crawford have been such a sensation without that horrible brown speck on her upper lip? I think both of them would've done all right without the so-called beauty marks. Cindy Crawford was known as "The Body," after all, and not "The Mole."

Some moles are deadly. I mean melanomas and other types of skin cancer. What you think of as harmless little beauty marks might be cancer waiting to happen. The only way to tell is having a skin screening at the dermatologist. A full-body screening. You will be naked, and the doctor will examine every last inch of your skin. But don't worry about feeling exposed. For the doctor, it's like looking at a Seurat painting from up close. All he sees are dots.

To excise a mole, the doctor can do it a few ways. Level it with a scalpel and cauterize the wound. He can use a "punch" tool for big or deep moles and sutures inside and outside the skin. Some try to zap a mole with a pigmented laser, although, for a three-dimensional mark, that probably won't help much. However the mole is removed, I recommend you go to a plastic surgeon—especially if it's on your face, neck,

---

*The French also like women with hairy armpits and Jerry Lewis. Go figure.

chest, or shoulder. Plastic surgeons are the best for cutting and stitching without leaving scars.

An actress friend had a basal cell carcinoma removed from her cheek, and the surgeon made the incision along the natural curve, so it's completely hidden in shadow. Good boy!

## ( Five )

# You're So Smooth: Skin

*All her life, Joan had "problematic skin." Problematic, because it had prevented her from ever having a boyfriend and going near small children without scaring them. But now, she was determined to get rid of the acne scars that had plagued her since high school and would do it without consulting a doctor. She knew she wasn't alone in this. Both Vanessa Williams and Jessica Simpson, among others, had suffered the pain of acne and the scars it left behind. Joan had heard that many people had fixed their scars with chemical peels, and she would do the same.*

*Twenty-two hours later, Joan parachuted from an Aeroflot jet into the mostly abandoned city of Chernobyl for her very first chemical peel. After she crash-landed on a little shack in the shadow of the nuclear reactor, the city's only remaining inhabitants emerged—a ninety-nine-year-old babushka and her nine-headed kitten, Ivan. The old woman immediately mistook Joan—who looked like a Russian stacking doll inside her gigantic silver hazmat suit—for a space alien with bad skin. Agents of the former*

*KGB were dispatched, and Joan was hauled off for questioning under fluo-*
*rescent lights that only made her acne scars look ten times worse. When*
*the interrogation was finally over, she immediately placed a collect call to*
*a dermatologist back home and vowed to come in for a chemical peel just*
*as soon as she was released from the decontamination shower (à la Silk-*
*wood) that she was forced to take.*

Go outside, right now, and find a baby.

They tend to hang out at parks and in carriages on the street.
Check out her dewy baby skin. It's perfect, uniform in color, with tiny
pores, smooth as glass, and soft to the touch, isn't it?

Now, apologize to the mother and back away slowly from the
stroller.

Okay, now go home, wash your face of all makeup, and look at
your own skin. Unless you've been a very good girl, worn hats, applied SPF 5,000 on your face every morning, and never had a cigarette, your skin looks a lot different than that baby's. Or your child's
or grandchild's.

A woman's skin should be a blank canvas upon which your husband, date, boss/potential boss, ladies at the club/bitches in the PTA
can cast whatever impression they'd like. If the canvas is splotchy,
spotted, lined, dotted, and dashed, people will form other ideas
about who you are based on the blemishes and imperfections. You
could be the first woman astronaut, a professor of marine biology at
Harvard, a mother of ten, or the czarina of good deeds for the Bill and
Melinda Gates Foundation, but visible acne scars, broken capillaries,
age spots, and blemishes will make you look like a syphilitic prosti-
tute from pre-revolution Paris.

As I'm one of those women who would take a punch to the jaw in
exchange for perfect skin, what's a little redness, itching, and crusting
when a shiny, smooth face is the reward?

A friend of mine once felt besieged by her freckles, like they were
a plague on her face and life ever since she was old enough to say,

"lemon juice." She was so insecure about her spots that she hardly dated and had only a few boyfriends in ten years. After trying everything else, from lemon juice to skin bleach, she got a deep chemical peel.

Her freckles are gone for good.

She doesn't miss them at all. It's a new face in the mirror, and she loves it. Men love her, too. They're responding not only to her beautiful skin but also to her confidence. She thinks she's hot, and who are her (many) boyfriends to disagree?

Another friend had terrible acne scars. Her face was like the surface of the moon. She'd walk in the room and the game would change from Spin the Bottle to Quick, Let's Break It! She was self-conscious about it as a teenager and increasingly so as an adult.

She had so many holes on her face, Tiger Woods used to play miniature golf on it.

We all know how easily deep acne scars can shape a person's self-esteem and world view and make them want to hide. But if you're always trying to hide yourself, how will you ever get anywhere?

Dating is a problem, too. Men do not like leaning over to kiss a pizza face . . . or pothole skin. They want a woman whose face, and intentions, are clear and smooth.

Anyway, happy ending to the story, she got laser resurfacing, and now her skin is as smooth as a baby's tush. She happens to be a well-known socialite who I always thought was way nicer than she should be. I asked her once, "Why are you so nice?" She said, "I was an ugly kid, the butt of a lot of jokes." Well, now she's kind *and* gorgeous, so the peel worked out perfectly.

By the way, with her glorious new skin, she attracted and married an extremely wealthy man. Which might be another reason she's so damn happy.

Psychologically and literally speaking, fresh new skin is a fresh new start. It's a do-over . . . and life doesn't hand you many of those. So take them when you get the chance.

The best current ways to correct skin problems are, in order of their popularity, **chemical peels** (burning away layers of bad skin, or chemical exfoliation), **microdermabrasion** (sanding them away, or mechanical exfoliation), and **laser peels** (zapping away bad skin on the whole face, or going after just problem spots, or photo exfoliation). And, in a special category, **radiothermoplasty**, or using radio waves to tighten the skin. Starting with . . .

# Chemical Peels

As you might expect, a chemical peel involves putting a chemical on your face, which makes the top layers peel off, revealing undamaged and unblemished skin underneath.

In 2007, over a million people had their skin peeled. The treatment comes in three different peel levels: shallow, medium, and deep.

## Shallow Peel

A superficial peel is for women with only minor complaints about small acne scars (not craters), lines (not trenches), some splotches, pimples, or redness. It won't iron out deep wrinkles. You won't wake up with the skin of your five-year-old niece. You will get a dewy glow, even out your skin tone, and see fewer lines and holes. Your doctor or dermatologist will recommend the specific chemical concoction based on how your skin looks and feels.

His choices may include: 1) alphahydroxy acids, and 2) betahydroxy acids. Alpha always sounds better to me than beta. (Maybe because alpha comes first.)

**Alphahydroxy acids** (AHA) are made from food, including glycolic acid, which is from sugar cane. Lactic acid is made from sour milk and fermented yogurt. Hey, don't be too quick to rule it out on disgustingness. Ancient Egyptians—history's first beauty junkies—took milk baths for good reason.

**Betahydroxy acids** (BHA) are made of salicylic acid. They're also found in aspirin and beauty products like skin toners.

These chemicals are so mild, you'll find them in over-the-counter cleansers and scrubs and masks. What you'll get at the doctor's office is a stronger version of the same stuff. The way it works: The acids damage the epidermal layer of skin, which will peel away, revealing new, healthy skin. It also steps up collagen and elastin production in the dermis, making your face clearer, firmer, and springier.

**Rx:** Most likely, your doctor will have you use a retinoic cream (Retin-A, for example) for a few weeks prior to getting a peel. The retinoic cream acts like a primer before you paint to guarantee that the color (or in this case, the acid) goes on smoothly and uniformly.

What happens at the appointment? When you go in for the peel, your face will be cleaned. No numbing agent is needed; you'll feel only light stinging or burning. The doctor will sponge the acid all over your face, or just where you want it. The chemicals seep into the epidermis (the top layers of skin) for fifteen minutes, and then it'll be removed or neutralized. Start to finish, the procedure takes half an hour. You'll walk out a bit red. You won't need ointment immediately, but you should use the moisturizer your doctor tells you to—and only that one.

Warning: I had a friend who decided she knew best and added all kinds of holistic moisturizers to her recently acid-peeled skin and ended up with horrible infections and permanent scars.

The peeling part comes next. Over the next two weeks, your skin will flake away. Since the peel didn't go that deep, the flaking isn't so bad, no worse than what happens after a mild sunburn.

You won't frighten small children and no one will scream, "Leper!" at you.

There is no downtime with shallow peels. You can go back immediately to doing whatever it is you do. After three weeks, the peel results are as good as they're going to be. If you like the glow, but want to see more textural improvement, get another peel. People often have a series of three to five light peels, spaced a month apart, to reach their goals. If you're pleased, get on with your rejuvenated life.

Just remember to use SPF every day: Peeled skin burns more easily.

**$:** Shallow office peels start at $100 and go up to $300.

## Medium Peel

With a medium peel, you'll iron out deeper wrinkles and acne scars, as well as even out skin tone. If you're blotchy and have dark spots or patches, a medium peel (or two, or three) might be just the ticket. It also gets rid of pre-cancerous lesions on surface skin. The bad news: There is longer down time, more peeling, and increased pain.

The main acid used for a medium peel is called **trichloroacetic acid** (TCA). You might be familiar with it as a wart remover. Sometimes TCA is combined with glycolic acid (made from sugar cane) or Jessner's solution, another mild acid.

After your doctor gets a look at your face, he will decide how strong to mix his peel cocktail, using between 5 and 40 percent TCA. The higher percentage, the deeper the peel (and stronger side effects). This peel does affect pigmentation, so it's recommended for the fair-skinned. If you're darker than an olive complexion, this peel might cause hyperpigmentation, aka dark patches.

**Rx:** You'll probably have a pre-peel regimen of Retin-A, and possibly antibiotics to prevent infection during the peeling stage. At the appointment, your face will be thoroughly cleaned. Then the doctor sponges the TCA solution on your whole face or just parts as needed. The solution will stay on for fifteen minutes, more or less, penetrating layers deeper than an AHA peel.

The epidermis itself has five layers—the stratum comium, stratum licidum, stratum granulosum, stratum spinosum, and stratum basale—on top of the dermis, or deep layer of skin containing connective tissues, collagen, and elastin. A medium peel can seep through the strata of the epidermis, all the way into the upper part of the dermis, aka the papillary dermis. The damage is so profound that the skin on top will frost, or turn white. Your doctor will watch the frosting process. When you're white enough, he'll remove or neutralize the peel.

You'll continue to frost, though, for about half an hour. Just don't look in the mirror! When the whiteness fades, you'll turn red. Really red, like a bad burn. You might also swell and feel painfully raw. The doctor will spread some protective gel on your skin, give you a pain pill prescription, and send you home.

During the healing stage, keep your skin moist and stay indoors. No sun exposure at all! If you must leave the house during daylight hours, wear doctor-approved SPF 30 lotion, wear a big hat, carry an umbrella, or wear a veil.

You probably won't want to go outside anyway. You'll be really red, and then you'll peel, crust, and flake. Whatever you do, do not pick! Let it slough off on its own.

After ten days, the damaged skin will be gone, and your new skin will shine through. It'll stay reddish for a month, but nothing a little foundation and/or powder won't hide. All that ravaging of the dermis will stimulate new collagen and elastic growth, so you'll see a new firmness, too, over time, to go with the uniform tone, smooth surface, and radiant glow.

**$$:** Often, one medium peel is enough. Just as often, peelers go back for more. Each round will cost from $500 to $1,200.

## Deep Peel

Phenol peels go deep. As deep as you *can* go, actually, seeping into the mid-dermis. These peels are for seriously sun-damaged or scarred people only! According to New York–based dermatologist Dr. Shilesh Iyer, "Phenol peels aren't done very much these days. It's a very aggressive approach but with big risks."

For example, after you have a deep peel, your skin will lose its ability to tan. It'll be paler than the skin of your neck and the results are permanent. You will always have a moon goddess glow. For this reason, dark-skinned people are not candidates for phenol peels.

The appeal of deep peels? If you can find a well-trained doctor with a lot of experience, a deep peel will smooth your skin perfectly in one shot. Not only will you kiss freckles and age spots goodbye, you'll peel away decades of wrinkles and lines, as well as pre-cancerous lesions that aren't even visible on the surface of the skin yet. It's the U-bomb of peels.

You will destroy everything, and there's no going back.

Phenol is also an acid, formerly known as carbolic acid. In other forms, it's an antiseptic, an herbicide, and a synthetic resin. It's toxic in high doses. Fortunately, your board-certified dermatologist or plastic surgeon is well aware of the proper concentration for his mixture. Usually, phenol isn't taken straight up or neat. It's mixed with water, olive oil, or croton oil for better seepage into the skin.

**Rx:** You won't pre-treat with Retin-A this time, although you will probably go on antibiotics and antiviral medications before the peel and keep taking them for the early stages of healing. You'll arrive at the appointed hour at the doc's office. He'll clean your skin, apply a topical or local anesthetic. You'll need it. The burning and stinging sensation is intense with a deep peel.

If you are offered sedation, take it. I'd take it for a manicure, and you definitely want it for a major peel.

The doctor will paint on the phenol solution. Then, it sinks through five layers of epidermis, through the papillary dermis and into the lower or reticular dermis. But just remember: no pain, no gain, and all that trauma means significant regeneration of new cells and peeling away layers of sun-damaged and wrinkled skin. It is as close as you can get to a total skin do-over.

After several minutes, you'll start frosting, or turning white.

Keeping a close watch, the doctor will wait until you've frosted sufficiently, and then he'll remove or neutralize the peel.

It could be up to half an hour. You'll continue to frost for an hour, even after the peel is cleaned off. After the white stage, you'll swell and turn red. The doctor will slather you with gel or Vaseline. You'll be bandaged, loaded up on pain meds, and sent home with the escort of your choice.

After a deep peel, you shouldn't walk out by yourself. You've been sedated, and you have a bright red face that will stop traffic. The peeling and crusting will begin in a day, and it'll keep going for about nine more. You'll have all the discomfort you would if you had a bad, bad sunburn—which is exactly what you've had. Once all the skin has sloughed off, you'll still be red, decreasingly so, for up to six months. By that time, you'll have smooth skin, new firmness, and even tone due to the massive cell regeneration, collagen growth, and pigment bleaching.

As I said, with deep peels, the results are permanent. So are the changes in your lifestyle. You can never again leave the house without SPF 15 thickly applied to your face. If so, you will sizzle.

**$$$:** The phenol peel is riskier and therefore pricier. Expect to pay between $800 and $1,500. Unlike the shallow and medium peels, however, a deep peel is a one-time expense.

### Give Me a Retin-A!

Tretinoin or retinoin, otherwise known as the prescription drug Retin-A, is an acid form of Vitamin A. It's used as a preliminary peel treatment to thin the outer layer of the epidermis, and thicken layers below. This helps chemical peels penetrate evenly on top, while simultaneously stimulating collagen production in the deeper layers.

As if that were the only application for Retin-A! It's the wonder drug for the complexion. You name the affliction, Retin-A can fix it.

**Pimples?** Retin-A is their nemesis. It unplugs blackheads and whiteheads, prevents oil buildup and breakouts. Caveat: You have to use it every day for seven weeks to see a benefit. But what's seven weeks in the grand scheme? A hiccup.

**Wrinkles?** Retin-A is the ultimate exfoliant. It gently softens your skin's texture, smoothing over fine lines in the process.

**Sun damage?** This stuff is great for correcting sun-related hyperpigmentation. In other words, farewell freckles.

**Hair loss?** As an exfoliant, it keeps the skin soft. Soft skin lets other meds penetrate better. When Retin-A is used in conjunction with minoxidil, the follicle stimulator, hair starts springing out of the scalp like flowers in May.

You'll have to get a prescription from a doctor. Shouldn't be too hard. For a year's worth of wonder cream, you'll spend $600 to $1,000. Your insurance company might cover it. Apply Retin-A at night, after washing and toning your face. Since you'll be extra sensitive to sun and dryness when using Retin-A, use an SPF 15 moisturizer every morning. You might break out at first, but after two weeks, your skin should settle down and start repairing itself.

# Microdermabrasion

After chemical peels, microdermabrasion, or mechanical exfoliation, is the second most popular method of skin resurfacing. Almost 900,000 people had it done in 2007 to improve the overall texture of their skin.

To understand how it works, imagine a seventeen-year-old idiot got drunk on Budweiser and spray-painted the word "balls" on the school wall. The next day, the janitor erased the offending graffiti with a sandblaster, a high-pressure hose that sprays a mix of sand and water, blasting the paint off the concrete wall.

If your skin were that wall, microdermabrasion gets the "balls" off your face. Only, the procedure doesn't use a hose, but a wand. And the abrasive element isn't sand, but crystals or, for fancypants, diamonds.

Used on the face and neck to blast away acne, age spots, shallow wrinkles, embossed or raised scars (as opposed to depressed acne marks), microdermabrasion can also reduce the size of your pores. Pores are funnel-shaped. The wide part of the funnel, what you're looking into when you inspect your pores, is blasted down to a narrower circumference, making pores appear smaller.

Microdermabrasion would give you the equivalent results of a superficial chemical peel. You would choose one over the other based on a combination of factors to discuss with your doctor, including acne, redness, skin pigmentation, and texture.

"There are nuances that require a doctor's evaluation," warned Iyer. "Choosing the right technology for the right person and condition isn't only a science. It's an art." You might read this description and have your heart set on mechanical exfoliation, but if a doctor recommends another approach for your individual case, be flexible. Unless you've been to medical school, your doctor knows better than you which method is right.

**Rx:** At your treatment (and, be warned, you might want to have a series of them), the doctor will clean your face, put some goggles over your eyes, and then pass a wand over your skin that pelts the outmost layer of epidermis, the stratum corneum, with a pressurized shower of fine crystals. The wand also has suction power, vacuuming away spent crystals, along with the dislodged layer of dead skin. It's machine-assisted, hard-core exfoliation.

It'll take only half an hour, forty-five minutes tops. No anesthesia needed. I'd describe the sensation as painless, even pleasant. And when it's all over, you'll have a smooth, clear glow.

You'll be red, like you fell asleep on the porch in the sun. That can be your explanation if you need one. Resume normal activity immediately. It's no different—recovery- and risk-wise—than getting a facial. Moisturizers and creams are a must during recovery. Although you'll be red for a few days, you won't flake and crust as you would after a chemical peel.

What's the rub with microdermabrasion? It's a longtime commitment. You'll need multiple treatments, at increasingly spaced intervals, to maintain the soft texture and even tone you've become accustomed to.

It's skin-treatment crack: feels good, gives you an immediate rush, and then you have to go back again and again.

**$$:** A single treatment will cost you between $75 and $200. Once a month for a year? Make that between $900 and $2,400.

## Laser Peels

This is the third most popular way to get smooth, spotless skin. Nearly 350,000 people had laser skin resurfacing in 2007. The process, in a flash, is all about light and heat. The laser is a light beam that heats the surface skin, as well as the deep layers. When the surface is heated, the top layers of skin flake away. When the laser light is absorbed by the deeper layers of skin, the heated dermis goes into collagen production overdrive.

As you know, a chemical peel also flakes away layers of damaged skin on top, and stimulates collagen growth in the dermis. So what's the main advantage of using lasers vs. getting a peel? It's that the doctor has better control. A hand-held wand device is easier to manage than a painted-on solution.

**Rx:** First of all, which laser to use? There are literally dozens out there to treat skin. The gold standard for resurfacing is the carbon dioxide laser. "It's a long recovery period of two weeks, and you need a really skilled physician to treat you," said Dr. Iyer.

"You could use non-ablative lasers like SmoothBeam that don't heat the surface of your skin but do stimulate the collagen underneath. It's less effective on acne scars than it is on acne, although people use it for both. Somewhere in between are fractional lasers like Fraxel. It treats the skin in microscopic columns, leaving unaffected areas. That speeds up healing. The downtime with Fraxel lasers is minimal compared to $CO_2$ lasers, and shows fairly good improvement."

For sun damage, a good laser choice is the intense pulsed light laser, or IPL, which has a full spectrum of laser length and targets both brown spots as well as diffuse redness.

The process takes between a few minutes and up to an hour and a half, depending on how much skin is zapped. You'll probably take antibiotics and antiviral drugs beforehand and during recovery. If you're doing acres of skin, you'll get local anesthesia and maybe a sedative, too. Once you're relaxed and numb, the doctor will position the laser wand over your skin, and give it a pulse of light. You might feel a tweak, like a rubber band snapping on your skin, but you won't care (thank you, Valium). When the lasering is over, you'll be covered in ointment, bandaged, and sent home with pain meds and a friend. Let her drive.

In short order—a few days—the top layers of your skin will flake, crust, and peel, exposing the new, fresh, unwrinkled layers below. You'll definitely have pain and swelling for a week and won't want to leave the house during the leper stage for up to ten days. The treatment area will stay red, decreasingly so, for up to nine . . . *months*. Meanwhile, your dermis is busy making new collagen, which doesn't happen overnight. Once your color returns to normal, you'll be fresh, smooth, evened out, and glowing for up to two . . . *years*.

Since the recovery period is so long, why choose a laser resurfacing over a chemical peel? "Well, you can stay red for a long time after a peel, too," said Dr. Iyer. "A laser resurfacing and a chemical peel can give you approximately the same result. In choosing which way to go, it's a question of individual needs."

**$$$:** Laser goodness ain't cheap. For one whole face treatment with the gold standard carbon dioxide laser, you'll pay up to $2,500. Only fair-skinned people can do it. If you're medium or dark, the laser could cause hyperpigmentation, making your skin darker in patches.

**This just in!** The Titan laser is a brand-new choice for overall skin tightening that uses infrared light to stimulate collagen production. "It's a newish treatment of deeper heating of the dermis to cause skin tightening, without heating the skin surface," Dr. Iyer said. "Some people do well with it. Some have modest results. The plus is that it's minimally invasive, with virtually no downtime, no pain, and no risks, except the possibility that you won't see much improvement." It's a gamble. A big one. The cost is $1,000 to $2,000 per treatment, and you'll need to have two or three of them. The risk-free boost sounds good, but for my money, I'd take the guaranteed results of a surgical face lift.

# Radio Waves

A least popular method of overall resurfacing is called radiothermoplasty, otherwise known as Thermalift, Thermage, or Thermacool. The treatment uses high-frequency radio waves to heat up the collagen deep inside the dermis layer of your skin, while at the same time, cooling the surface skin, or epidermis. The heated dermis contracts, tightens, and spurs the growth of new collagen for extra snap.

**Rx:** The radio waves are delivered via a hand-held device that is passed over your skin in a matter of minutes.

The big advantage of Thermage is that, unlike peels and laser resurfacing, there's no downtime at all. The cooled epidermis doesn't burn, change pigment, or peel, although you will probably have temporary redness. Also, during the entire treatment, you feel zero pain. The big disadvantage? It takes time for new collagen to grow. A long time. You'll have to wait up to six months to see tighter skin. "Some people have nice improvement," said Dr. Iyer. "Some show modest results. I can't say who will benefit more."

**$$:** The price for Thermage is $1,500 per session. If you are one of the lucky ones, your new smooth skin will be long-lasting, up to two years.

## Out, Damned Spots

Often, total facial resurfacing isn't necessary. Considering the downtime of chemical and laser peels, women without major sun damage, lots of wrinkles, or severe acne scars are better candidates for a targeted approach to treat the small spots and splotches. Say, for example, you have a few age spots but otherwise decent skin. Why pay $2,000 for overall laser resurfacing, when you can, instead, pay $200 to get rid of the dots?

Since it's tricky to use a chemical peel on a tiny area, doctors use targeted lasers to treat smaller problems. "There are so many types of lasers. A qualified dermatologist or plastic surgeon knows the best way to treat different problems," said New York City dermatologist Dr. Shilesh Iyer. "The laser machinery is really big and expensive. What happens sometimes is that a doctor will just use whatever machine he's got. You have to trust the doctor to use the right machine for the specific problem. You can hedge your bets, though, if you do research on your own." Here's a crib sheet:

For **age spots or anything brown**, Dr. Iyer likes a pigmented laser such as the Nd:YAG laser or the Alexandrite laser. "We use these for zapping brown age spots, precancerous spots, anything that's dark," he said. "You zap the skin over the discrete brown spot. The skin will get crusty, and then it'll peel off. The laser feels warm, but it doesn't hurt." The process takes only fifteen minutes with no anesthetic. For a handful of zaps, Dr. Iyer would charge $200 per session. You might need several.

If you have **port wine stains, spider veins, rosacea, or broken capillaries**, Dr. Iyer recommends a pulsed dye laser called V-beam. "It's for all vascular lesions and diffuse redness," he said. This laser works on any pigment that's red or blood-related. "The results are permanent in that the redness is reduced," he said, "but if it's the nature of your skin to have rosacea, it'll come back in time. Also, you'll need a series of treatments, once a month for three to five months, and then touch-ups once a year." Expect to pay $300 to $500 per treatment.

## Orange Peel

I'm talking about cellulite. Between 70 and 90 percent of women over twenty have it. The other 10 to 30 percent? Are lying.

What is it, exactly? Cellulite is fat. Broken down molecularly, it's the same fat that's everywhere else on your body. It's not "special" fat, except for the fact that you can be broom-thin and still have lumpy thighs. The difference is location. Cellulite is made of subdermal fat, or the fat at the bottom layer of skin. Body fat, or subcutaneous fat, is beneath the skin. When you pack on pounds, you gain subcutaneous fat.

Since nearly all women have cellulite, you would think it'd be accepted, like any other universal body part. It's not, though, because it's universally ugly! If only cellulite were as creamy and delicious-looking as melted chocolate. Rather, it looks like a woman is smuggling cottage cheese in her thighs. Cellulite has only two good purposes: 1) it's a great equalizer, and 2) where would *Us Weekly* be without Cellulite of the Stars cover stories?

People are so scared of cellulite that it has actually been categorized into four stages—like cancer.

Stage I: Dehydration and other factors cause dermal blood vessels, collagen, and elastin to break down and weaken. This, in turn, leads to subdermal fat cells clumping together.

Stage II: The lax dermis allows clumps of fat to rise. Minor rippling appears on the epidermis, or outer layer of skin.

Stage III: The clumps float ever closer to the top layer of skin. Meanwhile, they grow a fibrous covering that make them more distinct and lumpy. Dimpling is plainly visible and worsening.

Stage IV: The fibrous covering grows hard, and the clumps literally push against the surface of skin. Dimpling is severe.

So, how to stop cellulite? Forget creams. If someone tells you a cellulite cream works, he's selling it. If he's got a study that proves it works, he's manufacturing it. The only cream that *might* work is Retin-A: It thickens the dermis. Thicker skin means fewer lumps will show through. That's treating the symptom, however. Not curing the disease.

Mechanical cellulite remedies use lasers, rolling balls, gyrating heads, bells, whistles, stadium horns. **VelaSmooth™, Dermosonic™**, and **Endermologie®** all pretty much do the same thing—deep tissue massage, along with lasers or radio wave frequency to improve collagen production. But remember, machine treatments are a commitment. Endermologie, which has FDA approval, calls for eight treatments before you'll notice any improvement, and the best results are after fourteen sessions. At $150 a pop, that's a lot of coin. And if you stopped after your fourteen appointments? The cellulite will creep back into your thighs. If you want to get rid of cellulite forever, you'll have to get treatments forever.

Even then, if machine massagers work, they only improve the "appearance" of cellulite. There is no cure for it. Not even liposuction gets at cellulite. Lipo vacuums out subcutaneous fat, not subdermal.

I'm sorry about this. I wish the news were better. Cellulite is tough stuff, and the world of cosmetic surgery still hasn't figured out a way to beat it. Yet. We're ever hopeful.

I guess what Benjamin Franklin should have said is, "Nothing in this world is certain except death, taxes, and cellulite." His portrait on the hundred-dollar bill is proof.

# Six

# More Where You Want
# It, Less Where You Don't: Hair

*Joan could no longer hide the fact that she had thinning hair. Her scalp now had more bald spots on it than the tires of a ten-year-old Mercedes. This problem could have been easily solved with a hair transplant, but Joan stubbornly bypassed a trip to the doctor to find a solution—which came (surprise, surprise) in the form of a cheapo wig from Chinatown made out of raccoon hair.*

*Nobody was the wiser, but every time Joan put it on, she got the sudden urge to tip over a garbage can and wash her hands in a stream.*

*She quickly discovered why. The wig, teased in an Amy Winehouse–style beehive, actually was a live raccoon that had stowed away on a Chinese cargo ship. (The creature had raided the captain's liquor cabinet and passed out drunk on top of a Styrofoam headform where it slept it off for the duration of the journey to America.)*

*When Joan put the wig on, it not only looked terrible, but, at one point, the little creature woke up and bit her on the scalp. Joan immediately called a doctor who, as luck would have it, specialized in hair transplantation. He assured her that any pain she might experience would be nowhere near what she would have felt getting the rabies shots.*

I'm talking about hair, people.

Men long to run their fingers through your hair . . . just not the hair on your arms.

They love to bury their nose in your hair . . . but not on your chin.

If men wanted to see hair on a nipple, they'd go to the beach with their brother.

Men love big boobs (as if we needed the reminder) for the same reason they like a hairless woman: they're attracted to any characteristics that are different than theirs. Men don't have boobs, so men are fascinated by them. Men lack curves, so they crave women with small waists and big butts.

Men have excessive body hair, which they associate with masculinity, virility, and an outward sign of the sexual beast within. In contrast, men are turned on by women without body hair. He won't care if you were born to a pack of wolves in Romania as long as you are shaved, plucked, or waxed as smooth as a cue ball before he sees you naked.

I hate to encourage male demands on women, but the guys are right about a few things: lots of body hair on a man *is* physical proof that he's overflowing with androgens, or male hormones, mainly testosterone.

Loads of testosterone = thick pelts of body hair and (in an ironic twist) a bald head.

If you see a man on the beach who is bald as the Super Dome with the hirsute back of a gorilla, you can assume the following:

1. He will never say, "I had a hard day. Just back off and let me go to sleep."
2. He'll be aggressive and ambitious in and out of bed.
3. He'll cheat on you with a $4,000-an-hour hooker from New Jersey.
4. He is Eliot Spitzer.

Incidentally, women with lots of body hair have more testosterone in their bodies than their peach-fuzzed sisters, and all women have *some* testosterone. The quantity determines how hairy a woman gets. It also determines her sex drive. Men are attracted to hairless women, but fuzzier ladies have a higher sex drive.

To confuse matters further, the higher the sex drive, the more likely a woman is to tweeze and pluck and shave herself nearly to death to make sure she's smooth enough to get a guy's attention.

Excessive hair on a woman's body—as seen by men, other women, and the woman herself—is unsightly, unattractive, embarrassing, and just plain rude.

Unless, of course, you're a member of Dykes on Bikes.

In America, the aesthetic ideal is for women to be stubble-free. A mustache on a woman is off-putting. Even worse, a butt-stache.

The last thing you want is for your husband or boyfriend to put his hand on your leg and be reminded that the lawn needs mowing or the hedge could use a trim. Or for him to touch you in his sleep and wake up in a sweaty jolt, dreaming he's in bed with Sasquatch.

You'll never guess when and where women began the practice of shaving to be sexy. I'll make it easy for you: where *all* beauty obsessions originated. Ancient Egypt. (Are you getting tired of my shout-outs to Cleopatra?) Egyptians were the B.C. equivalent of current-day Brazilians. The Alexandrians—women *and* men—were devoted to full-body depilation. Why? Well, hairlessness was next to godliness, especially when all of your gods were statues made of gold, ebony, and bronze. The Greeks and Romans also prized smooth. A clean shave (chin to testicle to toe) was a status symbol for men. For women, a hairless body was a beauty requirement. The hairier you were, the lower down the social ladder.

And it was good hygiene, too. Kept away lice, fleas . . . and plebeians.

In classic art from those eras, you'll be hard-pressed to find a strand of errant hair on any of the subjects, even in the crotch.

Except for a brief fling in the all-natural 1970s, hairlessness has been the modern American standard of beauty. Nowadays, hair removal is the preoccupation of women everywhere. The only place you definitely want hair is on top of your head. And there, the more the merrier. Big hair comes in and out of fashion, but men have always loved it. A shiny, lustrous mane is your crowning glory. It's also money in the bank, the key to success, fame, and fortune.

Just ask Jennifer Aniston.

Beautiful hair is also a sign of good health. A woman with bouncing, soft, shiny hair eats right, bathes regularly, and has good genes. Gorgeous hair can make or break a woman's looks. She could have the face of a dog, but put thick, shimmering blond hair on her head, men will pant.

Put a blond wig on a parking meter, and some man will offer to buy it a drink.

A woman could have a pretty face, but if she's got scary hair, men turn to stone in her presence.

Just ask Medusa.

In fact, Medusa might've been the only woman in history, or mythology, who wouldn't have minded losing her hair. As you get older, due mainly to hormonal changes, your head hair will get sparser. That's right, another fun symptom of menopause. Every woman will experience some degree of deforestation. One in five lose enough to get depressed about it. Unlike male pattern baldness, female hair loss is diffuse, a little bit all over. You won't get a receding hairline. But you might see more and more scalp when you look in the mirror. Unless you're trying to seduce Uncle Fester, thinning hair is not a turn-on. A three-inch part isn't fooling anyone.

The challenge for women vis-à-vis hair is less below the forehead, more above.

# Hair Today . . . Gone Forever: Laser Hair Removal

Why do we even have body hair? Humans have been out of the jungle for thousands of years. It's been a few million years since we were chimps and grew our own fur coats. Why not evolve away the vestigial covering?

Would you believe body hair's lingering purpose is to make us *more* attractive to the opposite sex? (The ironies never stop.) When I say "lingering," I mean smell. Human sweat contains pheromones, subconsciously detectable smells that waft off of our bodies and into the twitching nostrils of men. They get a whiff. If our chemicals are a match for his receptors, he'll come hither.

If not, don't blame yourself. He could be gay.

Hair retains pheromone smell better than bald skin. This is why we grow excessive hair where we tend to sweat—the armpits and the crotch.

Ever heard of a "whore bath"? It's when you use a washcloth and scrub those two areas.

By depilating to be more attractive, we're actually cutting off (as it were) one way to send hotness signals to men. Lavender deodorant smells very nice, but it won't draw in men like the chemical kick of pheromones.

Ah, well. We lose one weapon, and gain another. Beauty is about pleasing the eye, not the nose.

Which brings me to the greatest beauty procedure ever invented:

**laser hair removal.** These days, laser hair removal is the number-one beauty procedure among women under thirty-five. More than 906,000 people got their follicles zapped in 2007. Hair transfers are not just for men. Although only 20,000 women tried it in 2007, the procedure is growing (even if your hair isn't) in popularity. Reasons it's the best:

1. It WORKS.
2. It's permanent.
3. It's not too, too expensive.
4. It doesn't hurt too, too much.
5. No downtime.
6. It's an excellent party conversation subject.
7. People you barely know will want to stroke your bikini line.
8. You never have to see that crazy waxing woman who yells at you in Russian again.

## How It's Done

First, a quickie on hair growth:

The life-cycle of a single body hair (on your arm, chin, leg, pubic area, ass, anywhere but the top of your head) is only three or four months. Each hair begins as a glimmer in the eye of a follicle in the dermis layer of skin. Follicles are little sacs whose sole purpose is to grow hair, and drive you crazy with their fortitude. You can pluck hair out of the follicle, but it'll immediately start making a replacement. You can send an electric shock into the follicle (otherwise known as the old-fashioned technique called electrolysis), which slows down hair production, but it won't kill the enemy follicle. (Not one shock, anyway. Electrolysis will eventually stop hair growth, but it can take dozens of painful treatments over many years. Compared to the laser, electrolysis is horse-and-buggy hair removal.)

The first of three hair growth stages is called the anagen stage. This is when the follicle gives birth to a bouncing baby hair that quickly grows and sprouts upward, through the dermis, to poke out of the epidermis as irritating stubble. The next stage is the catagen stage, when the hair reaches maturity, and the follicle cuts it off—like a parent kicking a post-collegiate kid out of the house. The hair says, "I don't need you anyway!" and leaves the follicle, swearing never to return. And it won't. It makes a clean break from the follicle and its supply of blood, then moves upward.

This is when the hair sticks out farther and appears longer (it's the same length it's always been, but now you see more of it). Which brings on the last stage, called the telogen stage, when the follicle regroups after that ugly separation scene above, decides to try again, gives birth to a new hair, and starts the cycle all over again. As the new hair starts to grow, the old hair is pushed out of the body and then gets stuck in the weave of your sweater.

Since you grow a new hair every three or four months, a single follicle on your body can produce two hundred and fifty hairs before you die. Multiply that by the number of follicles on your entire body—five million of them—and you're looking at 1,250,000,000 hairs to contend with in a lifetime.

Incidentally, the 100,000 hairs on your head have a much longer growth period, up to two years. They also grow at a different rate than body hair, which is why they can get so long.

Okay, on to the miracle laser hair removal procedure. No pretreatments are needed. You'll go to your appointment. Take off the appropriate clothing. Lie down on the table. The dermatologist will shave the area to concentrate the laser light on the follicles underneath the surface of your skin. He'll smear a translucent jelly like K-Y on the treatment area to cool and protect your skin. You'll put on a pair of goggles (the little ones you used to use when self-tanning, before you stopped that unhealthy habit) to protect your eyes from the intense laser light.

The dermatologist or plastic surgeon will fire up the laser and then start zapping you along the treatment area with the hand-held wand device. The burst of laser light penetrates the skin layers and is absorbed by the pigment of your hair. The darker the pigment, the more laser light absorbed. Since the laser will be absorbed by hair or skin pigment, contrast works best. For this reason, laser hair removal works best on brunettes (dark hair pigment) with fair complexions (light skin pigment). Snow White would be the ideal candidate. Her sister Rose Red? Not so much. Laser hair removal is useless on blondes (that is to say *real* blondes). What matters is the color of hair under the skin. If your roots are brown or black, you can laser.

As the hair pigment absorbs the laser light, it heats up the follicle and damages it. Enough heat, and the follicle will be destroyed and never grow another hair. This is good. This is what we want. The catch is that only hair in the anagen stage, the active growth stage, has enough pigment to absorb the laser's light and heat. Since, at any one moment, a third of your hairs are in the anagen stage, at each treatment, you'll damage only one-third of your follicles. Damage, but not completely destroy. Hair growth will be slowed, but it won't stop after just one treatment. This is why you need to schedule six to eight treatments, six weeks apart. That way, you'll hit each follicle three times during its anagen stage. By the end of your eight sessions, you'll never grow hair again on up to 80 percent of the treatment area. And the 20 percent of hair you have left? It's thin and straggly. Doctors recommend you go back once or twice a year for a maintenance zap.

Some of you might think of all those sessions as a major commitment. An hour every six weeks for nine months? That's nothing! A commitment is once a week for fifteen years. In other words, marriage.

Immediately after you've been zapped, you might be a little red for a day. Use sunscreen. After about ten days, your hair will start to loosen. If you tug a single hair, it'll slide out—proof that the follicle has been damaged. Between sessions, if you have regrowth, don't pluck or wax. That interferes with the growth stage of the follicle. If you must, shave offending hairs.

The length of each session depends on the treatment area. Armpits can be fully zapped in five minutes. The bikini area? Ten minutes. Full leg, toes to groin? An hour and change.

In terms of pain, it hurts less than a waxing. The sensation is like a tiny snap, and you can smell the hair follicles burning, although you won't feel heat. Each time you go in, you'll have less and less hair—ergo, less pigment and decreasing pain with treatment. By your eighth session, it's practically painless.

## What's This Gonna Cost Me?

Most dermatologists and doctors charge by the treatment area, not the individual sessions. So, the bigger the area, the higher the price. For full leg, in New York City, expect to pay a few thousand for a package of six to eight sessions. For the lip line, you could pay only $300.

An at-home laser hair removal product has won FDA-approval recently. It's called Tria. As of this writing, you can only buy one through a doctor, and he'll train you to use it. It's not approved for use above the neck, but I'm sure women will just love to zap their mustaches and chin hairs with it. It's a good idea for women who have some laser hair removal experience already and need the unit for at-home maintenance zappage. Cost: $1,000, plus tax.

## Remind Me Again, Why Do I Want to Do This?

The rewards:

**No hair!** You can ignore your crotch all winter long, but how great is it to put on a bikini in June without having to worry about hair sticking out the sides like a billy goat.

**No hair!** Throw out the weed whacker. The superstitious game of to-shave-or-not-to-shave before a hot date is irrelevant. Your legs are hairless as an Egyptian cat. Your ass is as bald as Charles Barkley. Instead of agonizing about what shaving will mean to the date's outcome, you can spend that time styling the hair on your head, which could use the attention.

**No stupid hair!** A denuded bikini area is fantastic for your sex life. With no hair gumming up the area, he'll be able to find your clitoris without a map.

**All the time in the world.** A friend of mine used to spend half an hour every day shaving her legs and forearms, and ten minutes every night inspecting her lip and chin for pluckable stubble. She decided to spend the money, and had her legs, bikini line, chin, mustache, and armpits lasered. It took a year and $5,000, but she added forty minutes to each day of the rest of her life. She calls it the best investment she ever made.

## What's the Worst That Could Happen?

The risks:

A tiny bit of **swelling** and **redness** are typical, but they'll be gone in a day.

**Burning.** This happens only if the laser wielder doesn't know what he's doing and zaps you too long or too often in the same spot. To avoid burns on the surface of your skin, go to a qualified dermatologist or a plastic surgeon. Don't let some schmoe at the mall take a laser to your flesh.

**Hyperpigmentation.** Rarely, the laser stimulates the pigment in your skin, and causes skin to get darker, like a tan. If this happens, usually in darker-skinned people, don't worry. It will fade.

**Hypopigmentation.** Another slight risk with darker complexions: The laser light might inhibit pigment in your skin, making it lighter in splotches. Unfortunately, lightened areas will stay that way.

# Gone Today . . . Hair Tomorrow: Hair Transplants

Up to a few years ago, hair transplants were a men-only phenomenon. That was because no one wanted to acknowledge that thinning hair was not just what men had. They don't call it female-pattern balding. These days, it's different. The problem is out of the closet—or hat box—and is acknowledged as a problem, and science has come up with solutions. When the top of your head looks like a bowling ball, it's time to think about hair transplants.

I have a friend—herself a dermatologist—who got a transplant. They took hair from the back of her head in patches and moved it to the top. It took a long time, lots of procedures, and months of waiting before she noticed any change. It's been two years, and now she looks fantastic. She loves to shake her hair, which is now thick as mink. And you'd never know by looking at her that it's been surgically enhanced.

## How It's Done

Make no mistake, this is surgery. Whenever a scalpel is used, it's time to call the plastic surgeon. I'm not going to split hairs, as it were, and dwell on the blood and gore, although there is some with this procedure. Here's what will happen to you during a hair transplant procedure.

1.  You go to the surgeon's office, prepared to spend the better part of the afternoon there. In fact, be prepared to spend the better part of many afternoons there, as you'll probably have several sessions to fill out your head.
2.  You'll get anesthesia. Probably local, but maybe general. For a procedure that takes hours, personally, I'd rather sleep through it. But the risk goes up whenever you go under. It's a choice between you and your doctor.

3.  Once you're numb or asleep, your scalp will be cleaned. Then the doctor will decide which parts of your hair—usually in the thicker, back-of-the-head area—to use as donor grafts. Grafts can be round (ten to fifteen hairs), mini (two to four hairs), micro (one or two hairs), slits (four to ten hairs), or strips (thirty to forty hairs). He might do several slits and a strip. Or a round and a mini, depending on the area.

4.  The doctor will trim the hairs on the donor patch, and then cut it out—skin, follicles, and all. He'll fit that donor graft into a hole or slit he's made in the bald part of the scalp. If he's doing a bunch in the same area, they'll be in rows an eighth of an inch apart. In your next session, he'll fill out the area so it looks more natural and less like rows of planted corn.

5.  The donor scalp area will be stitched up with one or a few sutures. They'll be small and won't show through your hair.

6.  You'll be squirted with saline, cleaned, and bandaged. Your doctor might have you wear a compression garment on your head for a couple days. If you've had general anesthesia, you'll sit around for a while before your escort can take you home.

## What's This Gonna Cost Me?

It totally depends on how much hair is moved, what kind of hair you have (curly, straight), and what anesthesia you choose. A good range is $3,000 to $5,000. Per procedure. And there will be several of those. It's a lot, true. But hair doesn't grow on trees, either. And it's permanent.

## Remind Me Again, Why Do I Want to Do This?

The rewards:

No one ever again asks you to bend down so they can put on their lipstick in the reflection of your scalp.

Your hair might not be as lustrous as it once was, but you'll have more confidence in a convertible.

**Warmth.** We do have hair for a reason.

You won't lose hours moving your part from the left, to the right, or in the middle, searching for the style that hides the thinning hair. Now you can part your hair anywhere with confidence.

**Relief from self-consciousness and anxiety.** So much of plastic surgery is about not hating something. When the source of anxiety is gone, the daily joy and relief are tremendous. This is especially true about hair. Unless you really love hats, you can't hide a balding head under clothes.

## What's The Worst That Could Happen?

The risks:

**Death.** Remember, anytime you have general anesthesia, there's a small risk that you won't wake up. I have to put that out there, no matter how remote the possibility. As always, talk to your anesthesiologist to get his credentials and make sure he's totally qualified.

**Swelling** and **bruising.** These are two constants when you have surgery of any kind. The swelling will go down in a week and be held at bay by a compression garment. Bruising? Well, you won't see a lot of it under the hair in back. On top, the discoloration should fade in a week or two. Meanwhile, wear a hat or a scarf.

**Pain.** Your scalp will feel tight, throbby, achy. You've been cut with knives; this shouldn't be too surprising.

Alternatively, **numbing.** Pain here, numb spot there. Sensation should return—in time for your next graft transfer.

**Grime.** No hair washing for at least a few days. Think of it as a scalp oil spa treatment.

**Gray.** No hair dying for a couple of months.

**Butt softening.** You can't exercise for three weeks, as working out gets your blood flowing. Ordinarily, that's good, but in this case, your transplants might spring leaks.

**Celibacy.** See above, re: blood flow. No getting it on for ten days. Not that you'll be in the mood. See above, re: pain.

**Mad impatience.** Transplants require a level of commitment seen in few marriages. You will need multiple treatments over a couple of years, as you're moving only a few hundred hairs per session, with a couple months of healing between each transfer procedure. What's worse, the transplanted hair is going to fall out after six weeks. It'll regrow in another six weeks. But be warned, there will be a period when you look worse before you look better.

**Failure.** Some follicles won't take to their new location. Like moving a thriving plant from one location to another where it withers and dies, some of your transplanted hair will die, no matter how much you talk to it.

## Rogaine for Women

Can hair growth come in a bottle? Men have minoxidil (Rogaine) and finasteride (Propecia) to stimulate hair regrowth and thicken it up. What about the ladies? Is there a kind of bottle blonde you'd want to pay attention to?

Why, yes, there is. And guess what? It's for men. As you probably already know, Rogaine—the only FDA-approved treatment for women's hair loss—markets a female version. It's got a 2-percent minoxidil concentration. The men's preparation has 5 percent. In a 2003 study of nearly four hundred women, the subjects with the best results used the 5-percent formula. The only drawback is that some of them started growing hair out of their foreheads like Eddie Munster.

No kidding.

In those cases, the researchers scaled back to the 2 percent preparation, and the errant hairs stopped growing. Prescribing men's-strength Rogaine to women is considered "off-label," meaning it's being used for something other than what it was approved for. Do not expect miracles, sadly.

According to the study I saw, only 19 percent of women had moderate hair regrowth after eight months of treatment. Forty percent had minimal regrowth. As disappointing as these stats are for women, as it turns out, Rogaine—at any strength—works better and faster on women than it does on men! No wonder there are still so many bald men walking about out there. Before you go to the pharmacy and buy Rogaine for men, consult with your doctor first, just so he can keep an eye on your scalp.

And your forehead.

# Seven

# About **Face Lifts**

*With her smooth forehead, new hair, clear skin, and luscious mouth Joan was making many new friends, but gravity was not one of them. Her face was dropping faster than the value of the dollar (even in Canada). Joan knew in her heart that a complete face lift was the answer, but fear drove her to find an alternate solution. She saw an ad by the Air Force seeking volunteers to test the effects of G-forces on the human body, and so she devised a plan. Joan knew that the more acceleration she could tolerate inside the centrifuge chamber, the longer her face would remain pulled back and frozen in place. The stakes were high, but she was prepared to go the distance. A gorgeous tight face would attract suitors, and Joan knew suitors would bring with them orgasms and gifts, both things she enjoyed and looked forward to receiving from someone other than herself. Joan figured she could endure a little G-force for as long as needed if that meant it eventually led to the G-spot! Unfortunately, the centrifuge conked out just as Joan broke the all-time G-force endurance-test record. She spent the next hour bent over the toilet from motion sickness, which only increased the pull of gravity on her face. Disoriented, she stumbled off the base and managed to dial a plastic surgeon and set up a consultation.*

The face lift: It's the biggie—the lift procedure that pops into everyone's head when they hear the phrase "plastic surgery." It's the anchor—all other procedures are built around it.

According to a recent government study (yes, another waste of taxpayer money), the average man looks first at a woman's breasts, then her butt, then the legs, then the crotch. After all that, if he's not drunk, he will lift his gaze to a woman's face.

He might then recoil in shock and horror, no matter how tight your body, if you are a jowly hag with three chins and chipmunk cheeks.

Once a woman hits fifty, the face and neck muscles and the skin lose their strength and stretchiness. The below-the-neck muscles and skin suffer, too, with age, but at least you can hit the gym to tone your body. You can't lift weights with your cheeks. Blame gravity, sun damage, smoking. They conspire against you, causing droopage.

Droopage is not a medical diagnosis. *It's a natural disaster!*

You can either live with a road map for a face, or you can join the ranks of the 118,414 women who had what I like to consider "facial feng shui" in 2007, making it the sixth most popular cosmetic plastic surgery of the year.

Professionals call it rhytidectomy. I call it "Dear Old Friend."

I've had my face overhauled—chin to forehead, ear to ear—twice. The first time was in 1975. I mentioned this story in the book's introduction, about coming out of the operating room wrapped up like a mummy and seeing two women I knew with the same exact bandaging as I had. And each had the gall to say she was in a car accident! Plastic surgery was a shameful secret then.

Times have changed, and people are more open about it. Gene Simmons of the rock band KISS and his girlfriend, Shannon Tweed, got his-and-her face lifts, had them filmed, and showed the footage on his TV reality show. These days, if you say you're going in for a lift, your friends won't scorn you. They'll form a line to see the new you.

My first face lift was truly a major turning point in my looks and life. I'd made the decision to do it because I was sick of seeing myself looking tired and drawn. I was on camera constantly having my picture taken, and there it was, the starting of an uneven chin line, beginning rings around my neck, just looking, as my mother would say, "not fresh." I couldn't delude myself into thinking I looked fine—and don't think I didn't try! I'd pretend that nothing had changed, or that the problems were noticeable only to me. But then I'd see a publicity photo, or watch a tape of a TV appearance, and I'd cringe.

Not only could I see my turkey neck, but so could millions of viewers. Pilgrims started inviting me to Thanksgiving dinner. One fan sent me a side of cranberry sauce. It was depressing. Then I realized that, although I couldn't fix contract negotiations or change monologues already taped, my neck was one problem I *could* easily fix.

My recovery was relatively painless, or as close to painless as any operation could be. The only thing that bothered me were the bandages, which, in those days, were wrapped tightly around the face and neck. Every day, I looked a little bit better. It was like moving backwards in time. You know how it feels to grow younger? To see the sign of it in the mirror? It's terrific! Not just aesthetically, but emotionally as well. I couldn't wait to take my new face for a walk. One week after the surgery, I put on some foundation to cover the bruises and reintroduced myself to the world—with sunglasses and an Hermès scarf around my neck.

For all I knew, no one saw the difference. But I saw it, and, more importantly, I *felt* the change. When I turned to the side, I knew that my jawline was sharp and neat. What felt so *good* was to have all that annoyance and anxiety gone. All the worry and stress were over, done for, and the sudden absence of anxiety created a vacuum in my mind, into which rushed a new attitude and a positive energy.

That's when I realized what plastic surgery is really for: not for tightening, not for changing outward appearance—those are extra bonuses. Plastic surgery is for making *you* feel better about yourself. My confidence doubled. I always put on a good act, but we are slaves to our insecurities. In my line of work, I needed confidence to keep going, to continue putting myself out there. The face lift gave me a great boost.

Remember: Your face represents you. To help keep your career going or your love life kicking, you can take care of the one thing your boss, client, husband, lover, the check-out clerk, everyone, must see when he/she/it talks to you: your face, your advertisement for yourself. Your face is how you present whatever it is you're selling. If you're interested in making a change—in your career or love life—you can start by rejuvenating your face. Body flaws can be hidden, but you can't hide your face behind a veil all the time.

Unless, of course, you live in Saudi Arabia.

I'm not sure if it helps to know this, but droopage happens to everyone. Even Dakota Fanning, eventually, will see her face fall. It's unavoidable. As each day passes, the elastin and collagen in your skin are a bit more slack. Facial muscles grow lax. The fat deposits in your cheeks (the one place you actually *want* to be chubby) begin to sink. The effects are only too predictable. They are:

**Turkey necks:** the wattle of flesh under your chin that swings gently in the breeze or whenever you move your head.

**Jowls:** these pockets of hanging skin along the jowl line that make you look like a basset hound.

**Nasolabial folds:** the deep lines that run from the corner of your nose in a vertical line down to your lip, à la Fred Flintstone.

**Marionette lines:** the vertical lines that run from the corners of your mouth, down to your chin.

**Tear troughs:** the deep, hollow pockets that form under eyes. The only good thing about them is you can fill them with actual tears.

**Rhytids:** the Greek word for "wrinkles." In American we call them "Faye Dunaways."

Each of the above conditions is the unhappy result of fat deposits in your cheeks surrendering to gravity and skin losing springiness. A lifetime of emoting turns expression lines into permanent grooves.

## Kiss My SMAS

Okay, here we go. The **standard face lift,** the classic, the tried-and-true, the Tiffany, the Steinway, hoists the skin and facial tissue from ear to ear, cheek to chin. It also deals with the all-important jaw-line and neck. God bless it, and long may it wave . . . instead of your jowls and neck waving.

The standard face lift was first attempted in 1901—and, no, not on me—and it's been tweaked, retooled, and improved fifty thousand times since. Initially, the aim was just to tighten the skin, like pulling the sheets up over a messy bed. The big flaw with this approach was that yanking back the bed sheets is all well and good, but it didn't fix the saggy mattress underneath.

The acronym SMAS might as well stand for Saggy Mattress and Skin. Actually, it's short for Superficial Muscular Aponeurotic System, or the network of facial muscles and tissue. There are ninety-eight muscles in the face, and we use all of them: when we frown over the VISA bill, when we laugh when we see a gorgeous model trip on the runway, and when we experience every emotion in between. In a standard face-lift procedure, the surgeon is going to raise your SMAS. If he doesn't lift the underlying muscles and tissues of the face, you won't get the results you want.

## How It's Done

I never want to know the details of surgeries I'm having. I just tell my doctor what I want and schedule the procedure. On the other hand, I have a very close friend who wants to know everything that is being done to her. So, if you're like me, skip ahead two pages for the results. If you're like my friend, read on, as I run down what will happen to a face on the day of a typical lift:

1.  **Cut.** Can't make an omelet without breaking eggs; can't lift a face without making incisions. After knocking you out (definitely you want general anesthesia) and cleaning the area, your surgeon will make a part in your hair an inch or so back from your natural hairline. He'll draw a dotted line from your temple region down to the front of your ear, curving down to the bottom of the ear, then behind it, and along the hairline for a few more inches as a guideline. Then he'll make the cut using a scalpel. Still with me?

2.  **Peel.** Think of your face as an orange, with the skin as the peel and the muscle/fat/fascia as the pulp. To get to the pulp, you have to separate it from the peel. Your surgeon will detach or "elevate" the skin from your face—starting from the temple, rolling forward in front of the ear, moving down to the hairline behind your ear—using scissors, forceps, whatever tool he needs to. The skin will be pulled forward over the nose, held there with a retractor, to expose the SMAS of your jaw and cheeks. It gets worse.

3.  **Hoist.** Depending on your needs, your doctor might trim or remove some of the underlying tissue. Most likely, he'll lift the SMAS—the muscles and connective tissue of the face—using a needle and surgical thread. With a few

strategic gathering stitches—like ruching the bodice of a gown—he'll sew your SMAS tighter and higher. Thank God for anesthesia!

4.  **Trim.** Next, the doctor will pull the skin back over your face, pulling it nice and smooth. Once he likes the repo-sition of the skin, the doctor will make several holding stitches—at the temples, near the ears, by the hairline behind the ear. It's like using pins to make a hem before you sew it. Once he's sure of the degree of tension—if the skin is too tight, you'll look like you've been trapped in a wind tunnel—he'll cut away the excess skin and sew up the incision. It's not over yet.

5.  **Repeat.** He'll then do the same thing to the other side of your face. Now comes the good part.

6.  **Neck Next.** To get at the turkey neck, your doctor will make a two-inch cut under your chin that will expose the neck muscles: the platysma package. Holding the skin open with the retractor, the doctor will then sew the pla-tysma muscles snug. He might remove some of the mus-cles or lipo some fat while he's in there, using a syringe or a micro-cannula. Then he'll sew the incision closed. Done.*

7.  **Drain.** Your doctor might put a drain in for fluid buildup. If he does, it'll come out in a day or so (at which point you can take a shower). He'll also put your SMAS in a sort of sling, like a girdle for your head, designed to give you support and cut down on swelling. That wasn't so bad, was it?

8.  **Wake Up** in the recovery room, awash with relief and contentment, knowing it's over and that you've done the right thing for yourself. The whole operation should last

*You'll look great, and you'll be able to gobble again.

about three hours, depending on whether you had additional procedures along with the lift.

Often, women have crow's feet wrinkles filled with Restylane while they're already under. Or they'll have a skin peel.

I personally think that while you're under general anesthesia, you should do any little extra tweak that you can.

## What's This Gonna Cost Me?

Can you put a price on feeling confident? Is there a dollar equivalent to self-assurance? You bet your SMAS there is. For a standard face lift, the range is $7,000 to $15,000. It might seem like a lot, but that total includes fees for the surgeon, the anesthesiologist, the nurses, the facility, the drugs, the implants, the follow-up care.

Often, people combine a face/neck lift with a brow lift, eye job, laser or Thermage skin resurfacing, Restylane or Juvéderm fillers. (See Chapter 4 for info about those procedures.) If you get the full overhaul, three or more procedures, you'll be under for up to six hours and can expect to pay . . . well, it depends on the doctor! A friend of mine wanted a complete facial rejuvenation plus a nose job. One semi-top doctor gave her a quote of $100,000, which seems insane, even by Los Angeles standards, where another star surgeon quoted $40,000.

For face work, it's imperative that you consult with at least three doctors.

Study their before-and-after photos closely. Be pinpoint specific about the changes you want and then get their prices. But please, don't choose the doctor with the cheapest fee! This isn't like going to a restaurant and ordering the second-to-least expensive entree on the menu. Pick the surgeon you like, then question—nicely—the prices. Most surgeons are fair, and you'll find, in most cases, you'll be paying him what he deserves.

If you can't afford to pay for the qualified doctor of your choice, then hold off on the face lift for now and start saving. Put off your vacation this year. Drive around in the clunker for a while longer.

As I always say, better a new face coming out of an old car than an old face coming out of a new one.

## Remind Me Again, Why Do I Want to Do This?

The rewards:

You'll have **a feeling of rebirth**, of **second chances** and **new beginnings**.

You'll **like what you see in the mirror**.

Have I not used the phrase **"You will look ten years younger"** enough?

**A few weeks off.** You have a mini-vacation from work while you recover for one to three weeks. And you can't exercise for a month. Doctor's orders!

Once it's over, there is **no downside**! Only upside! In today's appearance-centric, professional environment, it's far better to look forty and be fifty than look fifty and be forty. Let the slack-jawed among your colleagues opt for early retirement.

## What's the Worst That Could Happen?

The risks:

**Death.** Any time you're put to sleep and operated on, there's the tiny risk of dying on the table. The stats on death by anesthesia complications are one in 250,000. The best way to avoid dying is to tell your doctor *everything* about your family history, drug use, diabetes, allergies, blood pressure. Submit to a lengthy examination of your whole body to be deemed fit for surgery. Have yourself tested for unknown allergies to latex and medications the doctor will be using. Make sure the facility is equipped with all the necessary life-saving apparatus.

**Disfigurement.** A harsh word. Makes me think of the Elephant Man or Quasimodo. There is always the possibility that, after the operation, the two sides of your face don't match up. Your right cheek may be higher; your jaw may be looser on the left. As Dr. Steve Hoefflin, one of the great plastic surgeons, once said, "Even a Thoroughbred racehorse can stumble." Usually, once the swelling recedes, you won't notice the oddness. But a chance of winding up two-faced is real, and not to be taken lightly.*

If you had an implant put in as part of your lift, the implant might slip or move. If so, it'll have to be fixed with a second operation.

**Nerve damage.** I joke about it on my Geico commercial, but numbness or paralysis is a possible outcome of any face work. Nerve damage is caused by a scalpel nicking or bruising a facial nerve. It seems miraculous that more surgeons *don't* damage them, considering how many nerves are in the face. But an experienced doctor rarely makes this mistake. Rest assured, permanent numbness or paralysis is extremely rare.† Usually, if you do have some numbness or face freeze, the nerve was only bruised, not destroyed. You'll regain sensation and mobility after a few weeks or months.

If you're anxious about this, talk to your doctor!

You're paying your doctor not only for surgery; you're also paying him to talk to you beforehand.

After death, disfigurement, and paralysis, what's a little **swelling**? Okay, yes, those first few days, you'll look like a pregnant chipmunk. But the swelling will go down a little every day. Eighty percent will be gone in a month. By six months, you'll be completely deflated.

**Bruising.** Okay, the first week or two, you'll look like Naomi Campbell's assistant. But the bruising will fade and will be completely gone by the end of a month. Don't sit at home, staring in the mirror,

---

*Even if you're *not* a Hollywood agent.
†like multiple orgasms

watching your bruises fade. Go outside. The fresh air helps, and God gave us makeup for this very reason.

**Bleeding.** Inside the face. I don't mean you'll be gushing blood from your ears or your wounds. Sometimes, a vessel gets nicked or doesn't heal properly, and a hematoma happens. Usually, it'll stop on its own, and the bruising, lumps, and swelling are just a temporary pain in the ass (and face). To alleviate the pressure, your doctor can suction off the blood through a syringe. If the bleeder refuses to heal itself, your doctor can go back in and close it up, but that will prolong your recovery period by a few weeks.

**Infection.** The face has great blood flow, so infections are pretty rare with this operation. BUT—there's always a "but"—infections are more common if you've had implants along with the face lift. If your body wages a war of infection against your implant, your surgeon might even have to declare a surrender and take it out. You can try again several months down the road. Meanwhile, to prevent and fight infection, you'll be given antibiotics. Remember: God gave us drugs for a reason.

**Pain.** Don't forget: Your skin has been cut off your face, separated from the bone, hoisted with a needle and thread, yanked tight, and re-stitched to your scalp. Now, tell me, honestly, do you realistically expect *zero* pain? Well, guess what? For most people, there is discomfort but not *real* pain. Your skin feels tight, especially when the swelling is at its peak. But when looking ten years younger is the result, most people are delighted to tolerate the discomfort.

**Numbness.** Until your face gets over the shock of surgery, you might have spotty numbness for a few weeks. If you still have it after a month, tell your doctor.

**Scarring.** A skillful surgeon makes tiny stitches, in natural creases, so they won't be seen once healed. Until then, only your hair stylist will ever see them, and he'll have to look with a magnifying glass. Makeup—hello!—helps to cover scars until they fade. By your one-year anniversary of the surgery, the scars will be, for all intents and purposes, invisible.

**Necrosis.** Dead skin or dead fat under your skin. This is the biggest danger for smokers. Smoking messes with your circulation. If you smoke for two weeks before your surgery and two weeks after, the blood flow that promotes healing will be stymied. If healing is stymied, cells can die and a big black splotch of dead skin on your face can appear. Also, if tissue dies under the skin, the skin on top will dimple and dent.

So, hard-core smokers: for motivation not to light up for a month, do a Google image search of "skin necrosis." Bleccch.

**Hair loss.** As the incisions are behind the hairline, rarely some of the follicles never bounce back. Also, the hair along your sideburn area, having been cut and stretched, might grow in raggedy. If it does, have the offending parts lasered off permanently. (See Chapter 6 for info about laser hair removal.)

**Disappointment.** Unless you're also doing contour work (a nose job, implants) in addition to a lift, the essential you-ness of your face won't change all that much. For a realistic idea of what to expect, go find a flattering photo of yourself from ten years ago. Looking like that again should be your ideal outcome. If you hope to wake up with Angelina Jolie's face, you're setting yourself up for disappointment. Also, a new look is great to attract men, but don't expect your pretty face to be a factor when you're actually doing it, though.

Most men don't look at the mantel when they're poking the fire.

## Mid-Face Lift, Neck Lift, and Implants

Sometimes, a standard face lift is more than a woman needs. There are some intermediate steps that tackle problems in specific parts of the face. For example, a mid-face lift gives a boost to just the cheek areas. A neck lift fixes loose skin in the jowls and neck. Implants strengthen a woman's profile if she has a weak chin, jawline, or cheekbones.

Here's the rundown on each.

## The Mid-Face Lift

A mid-face lift, or mini lift, as the name implies, rejuvenates the middle of your face only. Women who don't have long, ropy strands of suspended platysma muscles in the neck or jiggling jowls along the jawline are ideal candidates for the soft-core version. I think of the mini lift as a starter, like a starter apartment or a starter marriage: the toe-in-water operation for women in their early to mid-forties who are noticing changes in their cheeks and ever deepening naso-labial folds. The mini lift will take care of these pesky problems without much cutting or messing with your SMAS.

The procedure is done under general anesthesia. After you've been scrubbed and your hair has been parted, the doctor will make a little incision—a hole, really—behind the hairline of your scalp. Into this hole, he'll slide a long, thin tube with a light and a camera on the tip—an endoscope—all the way down from your scalp into your mid-face region so he'll be able to see what he's doing. Then, he'll insert another long, thin instrument into that same incision to tunnel around and lift the skin layer away from your cheek bones.

The next step is to pull your upper lip up with a retractor and make an incision in your mouth in the skin over your gums. Only a hole, like the one in your scalp. This second hole is another tunnel entrance. The idea is to have the upper tunnel extend down to meet the lower tunnel.

It's a meerkat village of tunnels under your face.

Once all the tunnels are connected, the doctor will insert a needle with sutures into the lower (or mouth) incision and sew the fat deposits under your cheeks higher. He'll use suspension stitches or the ruching technique. All this mending is done under your skin. He can see what he's doing because the endoscope—still in your face—sends images to a TV monitor, which the doctor watches while he works.

After he's lifted the fat deposits back in their upright-and-locked position, all the needles, scopes, and forceps are removed from the mouth and scalp holes. The doctor will sew the holes closed.

Then he'll do the other cheek, and you're done.

From beginning to end, the mid-face lift takes an hour or two, tops. It costs about $6,000. The recovery is shorter than a standard face lift, although you'll still have to wear the special mummy head girdle for a week and shouldn't do any exercise for a month.

In a few weeks, you'll look in the mirror and see yourself from ten years ago. You'll fall in love. You'll want to take yourself out to dinner and a movie. Maybe you'll get lucky, too!

## Neck Lift

This procedure is for women who are okay with their faces, but feel like their necks have too much slack or wattle. A neck lift alone can do wonders for your profile, to make everyone you know think you've lost ten pounds, just by sharpening the jawline.

The procedure is also under general anesthesia. The first step is to get rid of excess fat by doing liposuction of the area. For a place this small, it's not a major operation. The doctor will insert a syringe and extract extra fat.

Once your neck is thinned, he'll go to step two: tightening the platysma muscles, the ropey muscles that hang down and give you that turkey-neck look. To do so, the surgeon will fix the loose muscles with a platysmaplasty: he'll make small incisions under the chin to access the muscles; he'll either stitch them tighter with sutures or even use a scalpel to remove some of the muscles, thereby shortening and tightening them.

The third and last step of a neck lift is to sharpen the jawline by removing extra skin. To do a cervicoplasty, the doctor will make incisions under or behind the ears, as well as under the chin if you didn't have a platysmaplasty; if you did, that incision is already made. He'll then pull the neck skin tighter—but not too tight!—to get rid of hateful neck rings and any bunches of flesh. Once the skin is reposi-tioned, he'll trim the excess and suture the incisions closed.

The operation lasts two to four hours and costs between $4,000 and $15,000. The price range is so big because of the multi-step process. Afterward, you'll wear a compression garment, like a tight turtleneck, for several days. The scars are hidden behind the ear, and unless someone is looking for them, they won't see them. In a month, you can resume normal exercise and drinking activity.

You can even go back to work in a week, if you feel up to it.

The swelling and bruising are gone by the end of the month, al-though you'll see improvement in just a week. At that point, you can start to wear chokers and low-cut dresses, and start to show off the graceful swan neck of your dreams.

## Implants

Most of us are acquainted with facial implants. Done right, they can improve the proportion and balance of your face. And what a differ-ence they can make! A slightly stronger chin or higher cheekbone can turn a pretty woman into a classic beauty. The material used in facial implants is a silicone rubber. Silicone is the stuff in most breast implants. The implant itself will be custom-sized for your face, wher-ever it goes, be it the chin, cheek, or jaw.

For a chin, the doctor will make a cut either inside your lower lip or under your chin. Then he'll create a pocket into which he'll slide the implant. For the cheek, the incision is in the skin inside the mouth, or underneath the eye, or, if part of your face lift, the doctor will use the incisions he's already made. For lower jaw implants, inci-sions are made in the mouth. The pocket is created, and the implant is slid in.

I think we all have the wrong idea that an implant, be it in the chin, cheek, or jaw, can move once it's put inside the pocket. This is highly unlikely. "The implant pocket is a very limited space, just large enough to accommodate it," said San Diego plastic surgeon Dr. Robert Singer. "You use sutures to keep it where it's supposed to be. Plus, the body's normal response is to form scar tissue around it to lock it in place. Sometimes, implants do move. If the pocket is too big, they might rotate. If the position is not ideal to start, there might be some swelling and asymmetry. Also, if you have an injury, you can push it out of place. But an implant won't suddenly migrate from cheek to jaw."

The operation takes about an hour and costs about $2,000 per implant. If you are doing it at the same time as the standard face lift, add that time to the length of your procedure. Recovery for facial implants isn't too bad. With a jaw implant, eating and talking will be tricky for up to a week. The inside-mouth stitches will dissolve in ten days.

## Non-Surgical Options

Any way to get a lift without scalpels? Well, you can have wrinkles attended to with fillers or have a chemical peel to resurface your skin. But if you need a SMAS lift, fillers and peels aren't going to do the job.

Warning: You might have heard about a Non-Surgical Face Lift, aka Thread Lift, Feather Lift, or the Lunchtime Face Lift. Be careful! They're not at all what they seem to be. Everyone was very excited when they came out, but the results are just not so good. My experts tell me that the thread lift is a clear case of "sounds too good to be true." In fact, any procedure that's marketed as a "lunchtime" cure is probably going to be ineffective and a waste of time and money. A doctor recently told me, "There is no magic solution. Spin and hype don't measure up to reality."

Warning issued.

If you're still curious, ideal candidates for the feather lift are forty-five and younger, have good skin elasticity, no turkey neck, and are not afraid of needles. If the standard face lift is like buying a house, and the mid-face lift is like a starter apartment, the feather lift is a cheap summer rental.

Well, maybe a tad longer than just the summer. The results of a feather lift can last up to five years, or so goes the claim. By the time your face falls again, you'll be old enough/ready for a standard face lift. Call the thread lift a stopgap, a warm-up, or trying a face lift on for size without actually getting one.

The thread in question was designed by a Russian plastic surgeon in the late 1990s. Called the APTOS thread, it's a single fiber of plastic non-dissolving or absorbable polypropylene. Why APTOS? Well, "ptosis" is the medical term for sagging. The "A" is for "anti." Hence APTOS Threads, the anti-droop suture of choice.

It's FDA-approved, stamped, sealed, good to go.

The fiber has tiny barbs along the length of it. The doctor will use a long needle, threaded with the barbed suture, and insert it into the droopy area under the skin. He arranges the APTOS (or any number of other brands) in the skin so that the barbs hook into place, providing a support structure for the tissue. He might use a few threads or a couple dozen, especially creating a supportive net in the face underneath the skin. The threads are deep under the layer of skin and invisible on the surface. What's more, new collagen grows around the threads, making the skin even tighter as the months go by. The whole procedure takes less than an hour under local anesthesia. Expect to pay $350 to $500 per thread.

So, okay, a feather lift may be quick, easy, and inexpensive, but that doesn't mean it's right for you. There are risks to consider: the usual grab-bag of bruising, swelling, infection, and bleeding. Also, weird dimpling, asymmetry, the off chance that a thread will come undone and poke out of its entry hole, a thread breaking and half your face falling down, a thread that can be seen or felt under the skin.

In all of those instances, the thread will have to be removed, replaced, or repositioned. They won't dissolve. They're yours to keep.

## The Shark Has Pretty Teeth, Dear

Good teeth are more important than a good nose. Ask any character actor: the first thing they do when they want to look ugly is put on fake hillbilly teeth. I think teeth are even more important than a nose, in terms of your general attractiveness and setting the tone for your whole face.

To whiten teeth that have been yellowed or grayed by age, smoking, or drinking gallons and gallons of coffee, you have a couple of options. The first is **bleaching gel** made of hydrogen peroxide. You can do this at a dentist's office or at home with a kit. You'll spend more if you have the professionals do it, naturally, but you'll also get better results.

To do the whitening procedure, the dentist will put a retractor in your mouth to expose your teeth and hold your mouth open. He'll protect your gums with a plastic covering. Next, the bleaching gel goes on your teeth, where it will stay for half an hour, often with a bright light shining into your open mouth to speed up the whitening action. You'll have on goggles to protect your eyes. The gel is then washed off, and a fresh coating is put on.

You'll endure another fifteen or so minutes of bleaching during round two before you can take out the retractor.

Most people aren't used to having their mouths wide open for an hour at a time (except Paris Hilton).

Cramping is possible. Soreness for sure. But when it's over, your teeth will be two to eight shades lighter on a sixteen-point scale.

Or so that's the promise. I know people who've tried whitening, and they weren't all that happy with the results. For one thing, the whitening is temporary. Keep aging, smoking, and Starbucks-ing, and your teeth will be back to their old color in no time. At $650 for a treatment, it's a gamble. Professional at-home kits cost $400. Cheaper over-the-counter kits are as little as $30.

A guaranteed, long-term (fifteen years) way to brighten a smile is **porcelain veneers**. Before I even get into how they're done, you should be aware that veneers cost between $1,000 and $2,500. Per tooth!

And you can't do just a few teeth, or you'll have what dental professionals call "technicolor teeth." It has to be all or none.

First, the dentist will do some tooth shaping with scary tools to improve your smile as best he can. Then, he'll make a mold of your teeth, get an impression of each one to have made into an individual veneer, which is a super-thin porcelain covering. You'll have to wait a few weeks before the veneers are ready. Then you'll go back to the dentist for placement. It'll take a couple hours to bond each veneer.

Afterwards, your teeth will be sensitive for a few days, but you won't care. Your teeth will be perfect and bright.

When you smile, people will reach for their sunglasses.

## Celebrity Face Lift Ticker

The thing about face lifts: If it's a good one, you shouldn't be able to tell it's happened. The liftee should just look "better," "rested," and "more confident." If the lift is extreme or botched, you can tell in a second, such as the face lifts on:

**Mickey Rourke,** once a hottie, now a nottie. He's had the screws tightened a few too many times.

**Sylvester Stallone** looks like Rambo did a search-and-destroy mission on his face.

**Burt Reynolds** has, apparently, spent the last five years locked in a wind tunnel.

**Joan Van Ark** has been lifted more times than Lindsay Lohan's mini-skirt.

**Melanie Griffith,** in an attempt to stay as pretty as she once was, has, reportedly, had many surgeries, each one adding a century to her appearance.

**Robert Redford's** face lift was a bit of a shock. He should have been doing little tweaks all along and not showing up at Sundance looking like a completely different person.

**Donatella Versace** has started to morph into a platinum-blond Muppet.

**Janice Dickinson**, a former model, tells everyone who'll listen about her multiple operations.* Her plastic surgery is no big secret. Her face gets more severe with each procedure. She could open a can with that nose.

She could slice bread with her cheekbones.

Kissing her cheek, you could cut yourself.

As for me? My face has had more blades on it than a hockey rink. Last season, my plastic surgeon won the Stanley Cup—and that's good! He considers my numerous procedures his own personal "War on Terror." A war, he is proud to say, he has successfully won.

---

*I'm dying to hear the one about her male-to-female chop.

# Eight

# When You Care Enough

## to Send Your Very, Very Breast

*Joan knew a killer rack would attract men. She saw the way men looked at the Barbie next door and recalled how her own mother's money-filled bosom had attracted many a male eye over the years. Joan was determined, however, to get one without surgery. She knew there were alternative solutions. In high school, Joan had once stuffed her bra with old gym socks and ended up with athlete's chest, so this time she decided she would use facial tissues. They're hygienic, coated in aloe, and fill out a bra nicely. The idea worked, and a guy asked her out to a movie—a double feature of* Bambi *and* Terms of Endearment.

*Little did Joan know that from the moment Debra Winger was diagnosed with cancer to well beyond the death of Bambi's mother, her date would bawl like a baby. Joan's bra instantly became a Kleenex dispenser from which she was forced to discreetly and reluctantly pull her two-ply boobage just so her date could blow his nose. When the lights came up, the guy was shocked to discover that the girl he'd had at dinner, with a D-cup, was now leaving the theater with an A.*

*That night, Joan learned a great life lesson: a man/woman relationship is bound to last longer when built on a semi-solid foundation of silicone. The next morning, Joan rented the complete box set of "Baywatch" to do some "window shopping" and she then promptly speed-dialed a plastic surgeon to discuss her own breast implants.*

So Chesty McHooter walks into a room. Do the men there watch her bouncing boobs and think:

   a.   "Those jugs are unsightly."
   b.   "I wish she were flat-chested and a lot smarter than me."
   c.   "More than a handful is wasteful."
   d.   They can't think at all, because all the blood has rushed out of their brains and into their throbbing, engorged . . . eyeballs.

The correct answer is b., but only if the man is looking for an accountant.

Otherwise, it's d., of course. I know there are some men who do say, "More than a handful is wasteful." But I want to know what size TV these guys have in their living rooms. Given the choice, most men would gladly sell their grandmother for a fifty-inch plasma and/or a girlfriend with big ones. Men love excess: in boobs, TVs, cars, cans of beer, buckets of chicken wings. The bigger, the better. I suspect men say that "handful" comment to their A-cup girlfriends. And they might even believe it a little, until Pamela Anderson sits down next to them on the couch, and they can't roll their tongues back into their mouths.

Breasts make the world go round. Perhaps that's why breast augmentation is the most popular plastic surgery performed in the

United States. According to the American Society of Plastic Surgeons, 347,524 mammaplasties were performed in 2007.

In Los Angeles, you can't swing a Prada bag without hitting a plastic boob. In Des Moines, you can see them coming at you from two blocks away. The desire to bust out crosses all demographic groups: Hispanics, Asians, blacks, whites. All want more.

The love of a great chest is hardwired in a man's brain. It's an inborn preference, proven by anthropologists, sociologists, evolutionary biologists, psychiatrists from New York to Nepal, and Dr. Ruth. Men can't help it. Despite this common knowledge, detractors have their say. "In the 1920s, small-breasted flappers were the female ideal of beauty," they claim, or, "In Victorian times, women wore corsets to hide their bosom. Big breasts were considered low class and gauche, for wet nurses and chambermaids."

And, in those chilly Victorian mansions, where do you think the man of the house was sneaking off to in the middle of the night? Downstairs, with the low-class chambermaid with the hourglass figure, while the wife in her boob-crushing corset was sleeping off her laudanum in her drafty, separate bedroom.

At certain points in history, *fashion* might've preferred smaller boobs. But men? Never.

## But Why Do Men Give Thanks for the Mammaries?

1. **Big boobs look like a big ass.** Evolutionary biologists stole this theory from me. For millions of years, females of many species used to seduce males by sticking their asses in the air. Some species even developed asses that look like targets. We've all been to the zoo. We've seen female baboons' red, inflamed butts and the impatient looks they shoot over their shoulders at the males. It's

their way of saying, "Come on, get it over with. I've got a lot of shit to fling."

Humans evolved to walk on two legs—an inconvenient posture for genital display. Humans also switched from making love doggie style to face-to-face (or, as in my marriage, face-to-bag-over-head). Men, being stupid, were confused by the switch: "Where did the ass go?" they wondered. To satisfy the males' need for visual stimulation, our formerly flat, empty-sac boobs evolved into plump, round, fatty-ass-cheek substitutes.

2. **Hefty breasts mean the milk wagon has just rolled into town.** Since it's every man's secret fantasy to father eight thousand children by six thousand mothers, and not pay a dime in child support, they are attracted to women with enough of a milk supply to feed their infant army.

3. **Mommy.** Even if his mother didn't breast-feed him, every well-adjusted little boy was pressed against his mom's comforting cleavage whenever he was sad, hungry, or cranky. Well, baby boy is all grown up now. And whenever he's sad, hungry, and cranky—or whenever he's happy, frustrated, glad, upset-but-not-showing-it, scared, perplexed, bored—he longs to bury his face between a pair of flesh pillows.

4. **Men don't have 'em.** Greedy bastards, men lust after what they don't have, be it a Porsche, a BMW motorcycle, a fifty-inch plasma TV . . . or a pair of big boobs.

5. **Media training.** Men (women, too) have had breasts shoved in their faces since the day they were born. Since baby's first World Wrestling Entertainment commercial on TV, he's been conditioned to associate fun, thrills, and excitement with big, round boobs in bikini tops, and

nipples that could poke your eyes out. Have I made my-self clear? Men drool in their beer for an ample set.

But here's a caveat: big doesn't necessarily mean huge. Men love qua-druple Js—on porn stars. Where would our adult-entertainment in-dustry be without beach-ball boobs? But, outside the realm of fantasy, a man can't survive in proximity to such massive fun bags. How could he be expected to get anything done? He'd want to stay at home all day and play with them. Men have to eat! They have to sleep! They have to go to work to earn money to pay their wives' plastic surgery bills!

Alas, big definitely doesn't mean saggy. Women born with double Ds might look sexy at twenty. But by fifty, they're tucking their boobs into their socks and getting mammograms and pedicures at the same time.

One word heard often in plastic surgeons' offices is "perky." Perky is a breast that sways enticingly when you run but doesn't flop in your face and give you a black eye. Perky boobs stand at attention. Saggy boobs have fallen and can't get up.

The wonder of breast surgery is that any woman can buy big. She can even buy perk. She can have the boobs of her dreams, or as close to it as she can reasonably expect. The plastic surgeon's second and third favorite words are "realistic" and "expectations." Big, perky, realistic expectations.

Once upon a time, B.P.A. (Before Pamela Anderson), men might have voiced ambivalence about breast implants, calling them "fake." That was back in the day, when implants got hard from capsule forma-tion (more on that later). Since the 1990s, great advances have been made. Problems have been corrected. And attitudes have changed. Now, no one seems to care if big breasts are real or plastic.

Did Pamela Anderson lose a single fan when she got implants? Hardly! Her fans quadrupled in proportion to her cup size, and no one cared when she got a divorce and had her implants taken out.

Then she got married again and put them back in. (This is common knowledge.) People talk about her inflating and deflating chest as casually as what they had for lunch.

No one would raise an eyebrow if she had a pair put on her shoulders.

Then there's the case of a famous TV star whose wife refused to get implants, so he divorced her. Enter the current wife, whose boobs are as fake as her orgasms.

Women also seek out gallon jugs for themselves. According to California surgeon Dr. Robert Singer, women do it to regain lost volume after a pregnancy. Or for a self-confidence and body image boost. He told me a story about a seventy-year-old woman who'd always wanted implants, but her husband wouldn't let her. He dropped dead, and within a month, she was at the doctor's office inspecting implants like cantaloupes at the supermarket.

"The misconception about implants," said Dr. Singer, "is that only strippers and porn stars have them. Wrong. Women of all ages and shapes come in for augmentation."

Dr. Steve Hoefflin, a friend and surgeon, told me that, in his thirty years of doing boob jobs, "Ninety percent of the women did it for fashion. They want to look better in clothes, to feel sexy and feminine."

Body image, self-confidence, fashion, sexual attraction, whatever. Having a beautiful, youthful body makes us happy and purposeful—and that's fine by me.

To sum up, having nice-sized and shapely breasts can bring a woman closer to the two sources of happiness and joy: 1) nice clothes, and 2) men who can buy them nice clothes.

## Breast Augmentation

Remember the song from *A Chorus Line*, "Dance: 10; Looks: 3"? The singer was a dancer who had great technique but was flat-chested and flat-assed. For the sake of her career, she got junk added to the trunk and bunk. New boobs and a backside changed her life. She got jobs; she got dates. She sang and danced with joy. You, too, might want to sing about your implants! But first, you have to get them installed.

There are several different ways to do it. I'll cover each one and answer questions along the way.

## How It's Done

*Warning! I'm going to spell out the details of what happens step-by-step, from the first cut to the final stitch. The brave and curious can continue reading. Otherwise, skip ahead a few pages.*

Okay, then. There are four ways your surgeon gets the implant into the breasts, and all of them depend on where he makes the initial incision. In order of popularity, the incision locations are:

1. **Under the boob.** The inframammary (Latin for "below the breast") incision runs along the crease under the boob. This is the most common approach for augmentation because it's the shortest route to where the implant goes. The doctor will make the incision along the crease and then tunnel under the breast using retractors and a tool called an "elevator" to make a pocket for the implant to slide into. Once the pocket is made, he'll slide in either a saline or silicone implant, sew the pocket closed, and then suture the incision line with small stitches for tiny scars. The scar will be three or four inches, but it's hidden in the crease. Unless you're a nude model, no one but you and your man will ever see it. Next:

2. **Under the areola,** or the dark circle of skin around the nipple. If the areola were the face of a clock, a peri-areolar (Latin for "around the areola") incision runs,

approximately, from 3:30 to 8:30 along the edge of the areola. The length of the cut depends on the size of your areola and on the size and type of the implant. This procedure is for smaller silicone implants and saline implants of any size. Saline implants can be inserted through the smaller opening and then inflated once they're in position. The doctor makes the cut with a scalpel, holds the breast open with a retractor, and then tunnels into the breast with an "elevator" through ducts, fat, and tissue to make a pocket for the implant.

Once that's done, he inserts the implant through the incision into the pocket. When he sews you up, he'll take special care to make the stitches around the areola small for minimal scarring.

The periareolar approach takes one or two hours, under general anesthesia. The major advantage to this approach is the minimal scarring. The disadvantage is that cutting around the areola will destroy some milk ducts, but you can still breast-feed after this procedure with whatever undamaged ducts you have left. Downward . . .

3. **Through the armpit.** Called the transaxillary approach, the surgeon cuts into the armpit and tunnels through to the breast. With retractors and an "elevator," the doctor creates a pocket for the implant. Next, the doctor inserts the implant through the incision and slides it into the pocket. After adjusting the placement, he'll sew the patient up nice and tight, both inside the breast and where the armpit incision was made.

The operation should take one to two hours, under general anesthesia. You can choose either saline or silicone implants with this approach. Scarring is minimal and hidden in the creases of your armpit. A two-inch scar might be visible when you wear camisoles, tank tops, and lift your arm to hail a cab.

Unlike other methods, where incisions are made on or near the breast, you can always say of your transaxillary scar, "Oh, that? I cut myself shaving." Even further downward:

4. **For the truly adventurous, TUBA, or through the belly button.** An incision is made at 12:00 on the belly button, and a long tool is used to tunnel through the abdomen and up to the breast. Another tool is used to make the implant pocket and yet another special tool snakes an empty saline implant through the tunnel and into the pocket, where it is filled with saline through a long tube. The valve on the implant is sealed when the tube is pulled out. All tools and tubing are removed, and you're done.

   The doctor does this "blind," as they say, because it's done by feel. It's called transumbilical breast augmentation, or TUBA.

   Unlike the other procedures listed, TUBA can be done under local or "twilight" (half-asleep) anesthesia, so you don't face the added risk of being put out. It takes only half an hour to forty-five minutes. There is no scarring. No blood. No cutting of breast tissue, and thereby avoiding damage to nerves and ducts. Recovery time is shorter. However, you can use saline implants only.

Dr. Lisa Cassileth, a Beverly Hills plastic surgeon, says about 40 percent of her patients go for the inframammary incision. About 40 percent go for the periareolar, and about ten percent have the transaxillary. "You can't beat the areola incision for hiding the scar," she said. "Some doctors don't do this type for larger implants, but you can stretch the skin. I've put a four-hundred-cc implant in that way."

The standard inframammary or under-the-boob incision is the easiest for the surgeon, so you might be steered in that direction. Make sure the doctor is suggesting the procedure that's best for *you*, and not what's best for him.

## Questions?

Several points to consider before surgery.

1. **Round vs. Teardrop Implants**
   These are the two basic shape choices for implants. By round, I don't mean spherical, just round. The other option is a teardrop-shaped implant, for that anatomical look. One day, no doubt, other shapes will become available. "Right now, I'd say eighty percent of American women use a round implant," said Dr. Cassileth. "And eighty percent of European women use a teardrop implant. On very thin women, round implants look more natural."

2. **Smooth vs. Textured Implants**
   Some docs prefer to use a textured implant shell to a smooth shell. The reasoning? They believe capsule formation—the building up of scar tissue that makes the implants hard and dented—is less likely on a textured surface. Some docs believe that there's no difference, in terms of capsule formation, and prefer smooth implants because they show fewer ripples and folds.

   This is a definite "talk to your surgeon" issue and should be discussed before you get anywhere near the operating room.

3. **Subglandular vs. Submuscular Placement of Implants**
   A question you probably never thought you'd ever ask yourself. Allow me to define the terms first: submuscular

means that the implants are inserted between the chest wall and the pectoral muscles. This placement gives the implants a smoother look, with fewer puckers and visible wrinkles. Eighty-five percent of breast augmentations are submuscular.

A subglandular placement means that the implant pocket is over the muscle and under the breast tissue. This placement is especially recommended for boobs that are saggy and in need of contour (shape) as well as size. The major drawback with subglandular placement is that the patient might be able to feel the implant under the skin or see striated lines when she bends over, what docs call "rippling." This is less likely with silicone-gel implants. Speaking of which . . .

4. **Saline vs. Silicone Implants**
   First- and second-generation silicone-gel implants got the bad rap in 1990, when attorneys filed class-action lawsuits against manufacturer Dow Corning. The lawyers claimed that their thousands of wronged clients experienced implant ruptures and that the gel leaked into the bodies, causing connective tissue disorders such as lupus, fibromyalgia, and rheumatoid arthritis.

Now, any company that makes a defective product that causes horrible diseases like fibromyalgia should be held accountable and forced to pay off billions of dollars in settlements, as Dow Corning did. And the FDA should remove the damaging product from the marketplace, as the silicone-gel implant was.

But, here's the thing: the implants, and Dow Corning, it turns out, were innocent!

Since that era of fear and media pressure, the scientific community has proven that silicone-gel implants were *not* responsible for causing all those terrible diseases. Women who never had implants were afflicted by connective tissue diseases at the same rate as women who had the implants. This is not to say that first- and second-generation silicone-gel implants were perfect and merely misunderstood. They *did* leak and break. Ruptures *did* cause infections. The escaped gel *did* cause capsule formation—when scar tissue forms around the implant, making it feel hard. Thousands of women *were* walking around with half-moon rocks in their chests, some of them bumpy and deformed.

But women weren't more likely to die or live in constant pain from the leakage.

In 2006, the FDA reversed its decisions and has approved the use of silicone-gel implants in breast augmentations for women twenty-two and over. Why? Well, for one thing, the research vindicated the implants ten years ago. Plus, since the '90s, manufacturers have been tweaking their formulas. The third- and fourth-generation implants have new and improved shells that leak a lot less (formerly, 20 percent of the time; currently, 5 percent of the time).

Less leakage = less capsule formation = fewer granite-hard, deformed boobs = a lot more happy customers.

Given their tainted history, silicone implants still make a lot of women jittery. They go with the "safer" option of saline implants. Keep in mind that saline (salt water) refers only to the filling. The shell of the saline implant is silicone rubber, so you're still putting silicone in your body no matter what. The rubber shell, when you see it for the first time, will remind you of an empty plastic sandwich Baggie. It has a valve and a tube through which the doctor fills the implant with saline. When he pulls out the tube, the valve seals shut. The empty shells come in a variety of sizes, depending on your preference. The sizes are denoted by cc, a unit measure of liquid, starting with 150-cc shells, increasing in increments of 25 ccs, up to 400 ccs. A 150-cc implant holds approximately five ounces of saline. A 400-cc implant holds *fourteen* ounces. Implants bigger than 400 ccs are available in increasing increments of 50 ccs.

The great advantages to the fill-to-fit saline implants are that the doctor can get very precise about size and can micro-adjust to the patient's specs. Saline implants are also cheaper than silicone, by half.

The disadvantages to saline implants? It feels like a thick-skinned water balloon.

Just as saline implants come in a variety of sizes, so do silicone implants. The shell consists of several layers of non-porous rubber, with a filling of semi-solid silicone gel; since it's not runny like it used to be, leakage is rare.* In Europe, Asia, and some select practices in America, you can get what are called "gummy bear" implants that are filled with a yielding solid gel that is reminiscent of children's chewy candy. Silicone implants come whole, stuffed, and sealed.

The advantages of silicone implants are that they are as "natural" as you're going to get. Silicone implants wrinkle less than saline.

The disadvantages are that silicone implants cost twice as much as saline. Also, the doctor can't make micro adjustments, which is a problem if a woman has asymmetrical breasts to start. He can get around that, though, by using different-size implants (25 or 50 ccs apart) for each boob to even out the patient.

**Hot off the presses!** There's a new procedure that's being done in Europe, but isn't FDA-approved in the States. Charmingly called a "boob jab," it's augmentation via syringe. Instead of inserting a self-contained implant in the breast, the doctor injects hyaluronic acid (brand name: Macrolane) directly into the breast to add volume. The most that can be added is 200 ccs (about a cup size). Price tag: $4,000. The injections last only a year and a half, might interfere with mammograms, and aren't, as we go to press, yet proven to be safe.

*like a Depends adult diaper

## What's This Gonna Cost Me?

On average, you'll have to cough up between $5,000 and $15,000 for the boobs of your dreams. It sounds like a lot, but you could certainly pay more. I've heard of women paying up to $100,000, or $50,000 per boob (I hope their implants were filled with liquid gold). At chop-shop operations, the kind of place that advertises in the back of supermarket tabloids, you could probably get an augmentation for a thousand or two.

I'll say it fifty times in this book (can't be repeated often enough): *from cars to shoes to surgeons, you get what you pay for.*

A doctor will charge what he or she is worth.

If you go for a bargain, you might have to have a second or third surgery to fix the original mistakes, and that could cost more than if you paid the higher sum in the first place.

## Remind Me Again, Why Do I Want to Do This?

The rewards:

**Dynamic, perky breasts that stand up and say (in unison), "Hey, sailor! That's right. I'm talking to *you*!"**

**Confidence.** Yes, it can be bought!

**Relief.** Women with teeny or oddly-shaped breasts talk about the simple relief of augmentation. They'd lived their whole lives feeling insecure and deficient. They were teased, ignored, and depressed about their mosquito bites/fried eggs/Milk Duds. After they get implants, women talk of the relief of fitting into clothes, of finally filling out a bikini top, of just being "normal." For such women, being normal *is* all it's knockered up to be.

**Implants can save your life.** The story: In October 2006, during the Lebanon war, an Israeli woman was hit by a Hezbollah rocket. Her silicone implant caught the shrapnel. She lived.

Another true story: On October 2007, a Bulgarian was in a

head-on collision with another car. Her 400-cc implants acted as air bags and prevented serious organ damage.

Still another true story: In May 2006, same thing, implants as air bags, saved the life of a woman in West Palm Beach, Florida.

## What's the Worst That Can Happen?

The risks:

**Death.** It's incredibly rare. You go in for a hot body and come out a stone-cold corpse. It can happen before surgery (a fatal allergic reaction to anesthesia), during surgery (a heart attack on the table), or even days later, due to a brain embolism (clots form during surgery and take a while to travel from the legs into the brain). Plastic-surgery deaths get a big play in the media when they happen, especially to famous people. The truth is, death hardly ever happens. A good doctor will do all the screening, testing, and evaluations necessary to make sure the risks are all but eliminated.

**Complications.** After the surgery, the risks are infection and internal bleeding. For infections, you'll get a course of antibiotics, and you'll be fine. In fact, you'll probably be on antibiotics before, during, and after surgery to prevent infection. For bleeding, you might have to have the blood drained surgically and the leaky vessels zapped with an electric spark to seal them shut.

Chances of infection and bleeding? Most doctors say around 2 percent, max. The scarier complication with breast augmentation is capsule formation, the amassing of scar tissue around the implant that makes it hard and bumpy. No one wants breasts that look like dinged car bumpers. Since implant technology has improved, and silicone leakages are minimal, the chances of capsule formation happening are way down but not out. Doctors put it in the 5 to 20 percent range.

Should your boobs turn hard or look dented, you'll have to have . . .

**Repeat Surgery.** Going under the knife again would be a necessary evil to remove capsule formation (via scraping it off), to replace a ruptured shell or a leaky implant, and to drain or stop excessive bleeding. You might need a second surgery to correct asymmetrical breasts, should one look bigger than the other, or bad placement of the implant(s) when one is higher, say, than the other.

Often, doctors won't charge you for fixing their own mistakes. (Ask if your surgeon is a fixer-upper during your screening process.) But you'll still have to pay the price for repeat surgery in time, energy, pain, and inconvenience. Also, be aware that implants are likely to get tiny ruptures over time.

The average shelf life of a saline or silicone implant is ten years. You might get lucky, and your implants might last forever, or they might tear in five years. Just be aware that having them replaced is a likely possibility.

You will have **scars**. No way around it. Ideally, your stitch marks will be neat, minimal, and well-placed. Depending on your skin type, the ease of your surgery, and the surgeon's sewing skills, the scars might be whisper-thin lines that only an obsessive-compulsive with a magnifying glass could find.

Or—the scars could turn out dark, bumpy, knotty, stretched, and large.

Bad scarring is hardly a crapshoot. When you choose your surgeon, examine the before and after photos with as much scrutiny as you give to the schmattas on "Project Runway."

There are creams and vitamin E ointments that can help prevent and treat scars, too, which your doctor can recommend.

Another permanent damage risk is **loss of sensation.** The doctor is cutting into your breast, after all. Some nerves might be sacrificed. Post-surgery, your nipples might be as sensitive to the touch as pencil erasers. The doctors tell me that, after a year or two, nerve endings revive themselves, and you'll regain sensitivity.

In some cases, nipples become even more sensitive. Five percent of patients, however, will lose nipple sensitivity permanently.

**Disappointment.** A lot of women go into the process with certain expectations of how their lives will change for the better. There's the initial post-operative euphoria. And then, once you've settled into your new body, you look around and notice that, although you love your new boobs, you still hate your old job, your old husband, your very old mother, your ancient furniture.

For other women, that boost in confidence (and bra size) is all they wanted and needed. The women who wake up and realized they're just as unhappy with Fs as they were with Bs probably should've been screening shrinks instead of surgeons.

Then there's disappointment with the outcome. Most doctors say that 90 percent of women are happy with the breast augmentation. Given the choice, they'd do the surgery again.

That leaves one in ten women who are unhappy, perhaps even angry. Disappointment can be avoided by going over with your surgeon how you want to look: pictures, computer animation, long talks—you're paying him to listen! If he's not a good ear guy, he shouldn't be your boob guy.

**Pain.** It's not a quadruple bypass, but a breast augmentation is surgery. Expect soreness (especially with submuscular implant placement), swelling, pain, and "incision itch." You can't shower for two days afterwards. You won't be pretty.* For a week, you can't lift anything heavier than a remote control. You can't exercise for weeks. They give you a boob-crushing bra to wear to prevent swelling. Be prepared to be housebound for at least a week, but I've found that recovery times are often shorter than doctors say they'll be. Shooting, sharp pain, tightness, bruising, it's all normal and to be expected. Sometimes, the "discomfort" (don't you love it when doctors use that euphemism?) can last for weeks.

**Rolling with the changes.** Your breasts change over time and due to pregnancy and nursing. If you got really big implants when

---

*Which is perfectly fine if you live in Romania.

you were twenty, you might not like how they look when you're forty. Err on the side of small when choosing an implant you will live with for a long time. Also, after a pregnancy, your boobs might inflate and then deflate. The impact on the implants? They might sag and swing around. "We call it the 'rock in a sock,' " said Dr. Cassileth.

A breast lift (see below) might be called for to correct that problem.

**Myths.** Breast-feeding isn't affected by implants, especially if you have the inframammary or transaxillary incisions. If you have a periareolar incision, some milk ducts will be destroyed, but not all. You will have just as accurate mammograms as before. And, no, your breast implant will *not* spontaneously explode one day when you're walking down the street.

# Breast Lift

Call them non-union members of SAG, the nearly 104,000 women who got a surgical pick-me-up, or mastopexy, in 2007. Although I can't confirm, my educated guess is that most of them were 1) over forty, 2) had at least one child, or 3) lost a lot of weight recently. Which brings up another oft-mentioned word in plastic surgery consultations—"droopy." Which is opposite of "perky."

Droopy, I'm sorry to say, is not Snow White's eighth dwarf, but rather the sad fate that awaits all women.

## Droop Report

Why do breasts take the low road? The same reason your jowls and eyelids and nearly every other part eventually surrenders to gravity: loss of snap in the skin and tissues. Decades of fighting gravity, combined with the inflating and deflating from pregnancy and breast-feeding leave your boobs with the ligamentary fortitude of a stretched-out rubber band. Every woman, even beautiful, rich, young blond ones, unfortunately will one day suffer the dreaded droop.

You can, if you're curious, measure your Sag Quotient. Professionals call the degree of droop "ptosis" (pronounced toe-sis). To do this at home, you need a standard ruler. Guys measure their erections. Women measure their breast sag. How? Easy.

Step 1: Find a ruler.

Step 2: Take off your shirt and bra, and stand sideways in front of a full-length mirror.

Step 3: Locate your inframammary fold, which is not hard to find! It's the crease where boob meets chest.

Step 4: Line up the ruler, perpendicular to the floor, at the high point of the fold.

Step 5: Assess nipple placement. Is it above the fold, at the same height as the fold, or below the fold? If it's below the fold, how much? One to two centimeters? More than two? If your nipple is even with the crease, you've got minor ptosis. One to two centimeters below is moderate. Two or three centimeters below, with a nipple that points south, ptosis is considered severe.

## We Have Lift

Okay, I'm raising the warning flag again. The next four paragraphs are full of slicing and dicing.* Not for the faint of stomach!

Okay, so how do lift operations work? Well, depending on your boob size and degree of ptosis, your doctor will recommend one of four lift tickets, all of which are done under general anesthesia. In order of severity of incision, they are:

1.  **The Crescent.** This is for women with small breasts and minor ptosis who want the nipple and areola to sit higher

---

*The kind you'll never see in Nobu's kitchen.

and straighter on the breast. You're not losing much breast volume here, just raising the nipple/areola package. The doctor makes two incisions. They are both semi-circular lines, the first along the top of the areola, and then another two or three centimeters or so above the areola. They connect at the corners, forming a crescent-shaped patch of excised skin. Then, he stitches the areola up to the top incision line, raising the nipple areola complex a few centimeters north. The procedure takes about an hour and is considered minimally invasive, with minimal scarring only on the upper quadrant of the areola. That wasn't too bad.

2.  **The Doughnut.** This procedure is for women with small breasts and minor ptosis who want their nipple/areola package to sit higher on the breast and/or to reduce the size or change the shape of the areola itself. The doctor first makes an incision around the entire areola in the shape and size you want. Then he makes another incision around the first one. The two incisions look like a small circle inside a larger oval. The skin between is removed, leaving a floating areola nipple complex, which is then stitched to meet the remaining breast skin, raising the areola up to four centimeters and tightening the whole breast skin envelope. You'll have scars all the way around the areola, which will fade over time. Stay with me.

3.  **The Lollipop.** This procedure is for women with larger breasts and moderate to severe ptosis. With breast lifts, it's all about the shape of the incision and how much skin is removed and stitched back together. A lollipop has a vertical incision and a round incision on top. The vertical incision is actually V-shaped, the wide part of the V on top and coming to a point near the inframammary crease, the nipple areola complex positioned inside the

V, like a circle nesting inside the middle of a triangle. The excess skin is removed; the areola is sewn to the top part of the V-incision, raising it several centimeters. The rest of the open skin is stitched together and to the lower part of the areola, thereby tightening the skin envelope. You'll have scars all the way around the areola, as well as a vertical scar running from the bottom of the areola straight down to the crease.

In this surgery, scars are the trade-off for having higher, firmer breasts. It's a decision. Which would you rather have? Sagging scar-free breasts or nice, perky breasts with some scars that will fade over time?*

4.  **The Anchor.** This is considered the standard breast lift for big-breasted women with moderate to severe ptosis. The procedure takes from one to four hours, and there's a lot of cutting here. The incisions include a circle of skin above the areola, a circular cut around the areola itself, and a wide crescent cut that removes the skin from the inframammary crease up to the top of the areola. The incision looks like a keyhole sitting on top of a croissant. The areola is raised into the keyhole and stitched closed. The remaining skin is sewn together vertically from the areola down and horizontally across the crease. The anchor incision leaves the biggest scar: a circle around the entire areola, a vertical line from the areola to the inframammary crease, and a scar hidden along the length of the crease. The scar is shaped like an anchor, hence, the anchor incision. Again, the scars are permanent. But so are your nice firm breasts.

If droop is only half your problem, it bears mentioning that lifts are often combined with augmentation. This

---

*Answer? No man will ever try to cop a feel around your ankle.

can be done in two stages or in one longer surgery. The doctor inserts the implant using an inframammary incision first and then moves on to the breast lift portion of the program. A combination surgery procedure adds hours to the operation, recovery, and, of course, thousands to the price.

## What's This Going to Cost Me?

Depends on which approach you use. The kindest cut, in terms of dollars? Anchor away. Paradoxically, the most invasive lift costs the least, on average, from $3,100 to $6,500. A crescent or doughnut incision mastopexy ranges from $3,500 to $7,500. A combination lift/augmentation will run you between $4,000 and $9,000, owing to the additional time and parts used in the procedure.

## Remind Me Again, Why Do I Want to Do This?

The rewards:

**Your girlish figure misses you.** And, God knows, you miss it! Remember what your boobs looked like, before the kids, before gravity grabbed them and refused to let go? Women get lifts because they long for the days of breasts above their bellybuttons.

**Confidence.** A lift raises your self-esteem as well as your boobs.

**Clothes.** In a word: strapless. And: backless. How about: halter? The gilded door of tight-breasted fashion will open to you, welcoming you with a cherub choir and seventy-six trombones.

## What's the Worst That Can Happen?

Again, here we go:

**Death.** Always a possibility under general anesthesia, if extremely rare. Since you will be operated on in an accredited facility by a board-certified plastic surgeon, with a board-certified anesthesiologist, the risk is all but nil.

**Complications.** There's a bigger potential for bleeding with the lift vs. augmentation, simply because there's more cutting and cauterizing of blood vessels involved. Rarely will a blood vessel start bleeding after surgery, but you'll need to be opened up again to seal the vessel and drain the excess if it does.

**Repeat Surgery.** You'll need this only if you have bleeders that need to be hunted down and sealed. Also, you might need tweaking if, once the post-operative swelling goes down, it appears that one of your boobs was lifted higher than the other, or if they seem to be different sizes.

**Permanent Damage.** Numbness is thought to be a major risk with lifts. But the vast majority of women who have some numbness regain sensation in a year or two. Some women, now that their stretched nerves and ligaments are shortened by the lift, have *increased* nipple sensation. In 5 percent of the cases, nerves are damaged in surgery to such an extent that sensation never returns.

**Scars.** The bigger the lift, the more dramatic the scars. With a crescent and doughnut lift, the scars are perfectly well hidden. With the lollipop and anchor lifts, some scars are hidden in creases and around the areola, but the vertical scars aren't. They'll fade over time, but they aren't going to disappear completely. If you get a skilled doctor, you won't wake up from surgery with Frankenboobies, but it will be obvious to anyone who isn't blind that something happened. You have to decide whether the breast lift is worth the scars. If not, don't do it.

Most women are happy to have high young breasts in return for tucked-away scars.

**Disappointment.** Head off a bad result by carefully screening your surgeon, poring over before-and-after photos of his work, following instructions, and communicating exactly what you want before you go under the knife. If he won't pay you lip service, don't give him your boob business.

**Pain.** Breast-lift pain can feel like someone's stabbed you in the chest with a knife, mainly because someone *has* stabbed you in the chest. Swelling, tightness, stretching; shooting, tingling nerves; bruising, sore chest muscles; it's the reality of healing. Your doctor will prescribe pain pills.

And don't smoke!

Wear the compression bra; keep the surgical tape on the wounds clean; don't lift anything heavier than a $1,000 bill. In a few weeks, you'll be hitting a tennis ball without being hit back in the face by your formerly droopy breasts.

## Breast Reduction

One hundred and six thousand women sought out a reduction mammoplasty in 2007. Many of them wanted a slimmer silhouette, a more aerodynamic appearance. But many also were after relief from a lifetime of lugging around a spare set of luggage on their chests. Physical problems can be caused by carrying too much bulk and weight in the front: chronic back pain, chronic neck and shoulder pain, poor posture, skin rashes, dug-in grooves from bra-strap pressure, inability to participate in sports (in particular, golf and tennis, where breasts literally get in the way). Emotional problems: self-consciousness, low self-esteem, a lifetime of being the target of gawking and teasing, deep frustration from never finding anything that fits, the bad feeling that people pay more attention to the breasts than to the woman.

And guess what! Male breast reduction is on the rise. Over 21,000 men with a condition called gynecomastia had reductions in 2007. This group felt like their breasts made them targets of ridicule. They felt like they couldn't take off their shirts or play sports without self-consciousness. They definitely did not enjoy looking like Dolly Parton.

## Now . . . How's It Done?

Here are the three ways to lighten the load:

1. **The anchor and scoop.** The standard breast-reduction
   procedure is pretty much the same as an anchor breast lift,
   except the surgeon tightens the skin envelope as well as
   removes excess fat and tissue. He makes incisions around
   the areola, and he removes skin in a keyhole shape above
   the nipple, as well as a wide crescent-shaped patch from
   the inframammary crease to the bottom of where the areola used to be. He stitches the areola/nipple higher on the
   breast to fit into the keyhole left by the excised skin. Then,
   he uses special tools to scoop out breast tissue and fat to
   shrink the overall bulk of the breast. Then he sews up the
   rest of the skin envelope, creating a vertical line that runs
   from the bottom of the areola to the inframammary crease,
   as well as a horizontal line along the crease. The round
   incision line around the areola, the vertical line, and the
   horizontal line create an anchor-shaped scar. Easy!

2. **Liposuction.** Male breast reduction is almost exclusively
   done via liposuction. Female reduction? Not so much.
   Sometimes, with smaller, not-too-saggy breasts, doctors
   will use liposuction to remove fat to decrease overall volume. (For more on the basics of liposuction, see Chapter
   10). A lot of doctors don't love this procedure for women
   because it can leave breasts lumpy and asymmetrical.
   Leave it to the men.

3. **Nipple transfer.** For really large breasts, a reduction
   with a nipple graft is required. Usually, with lifts and
   standard reductions, the nipple/areola complex*, with its

*Not one of Freud's theories.

underlying structure of milk ducts and nerve endings, is left intact and repositioned. If the breasts are massive and extremely saggy, however, there might be no way to reposition the areola/nipple complex without completely removing it and then sewing it back onto the breast, a "transfer," after it's been reshaped. Since the areola/nipple has been removed, all the nerve endings and milk ducts have been severed, and it will be impossible to breast-feed.

Nipple sensitivity will never be regained, although anyone who requires this procedure probably lost nipple sensation already from years of stretched tissue.

## What's This Gonna Cost Me?

Since a breast reduction is more complicated than an augmentation or a lift, it requires a lot of cutting and runs a significant risk of post-operative complications; it's the most expensive of all the standard breast procedures. On average, a standard reduction costs between $5,000 and $10,000. Take heart, large-breasted women! If you can prove that your massive boobs cause chronic back, neck, and/or shoulder pain, it's possible that your health insurance will cover part or all of the procedure!

## Remind Me Again, Why Do I Want to Do This?

The rewards:

**You can sleep on your stomach!** And **lie flat on the beach** without having to dig two holes in the sand. And then you can **run down the street** without giving yourself two black eyes. You can **wear a bikini** that doesn't feel like a straitjacket.

**Back/neck/shoulder pain, gone.**

**Under-boob rash** from sweating and never airing out the crease? **Gone.**

You'll be able to **swing a golf club or a tennis racquet**. I have no idea why you'd want to play sports when there's shopping to be done, but go right ahead if that's what you want.

You can **shop in regular stores for regular sizes** without having to have all your clothes custom-tailored. Your seamstress will never forgive you, but you won't care.

## What's the Worst That Could Happen?

Reductive risks:

**Death.** I'll say it again and again. Plastic surgery is still real surgery. Any real surgery with general anesthesia does have the risk, however rare, of death.

**Complications.** Some real worries here: bleeding, infection, tissue death from improper healing. All of these risks can be managed with good post-operative care or follow-up surgeries.

**Asymmetry.** I give asymmetry its own category with reductions. In this case, it's not only that one breast could be bigger than the other. They might turn out different shapes. If you had to have a nipple transfer, one areola might be higher or lower than the other. If having perfectly symmetrical breasts is a requirement for you, then I have to give a hale and hearty warning about reductions. They will probably look nearly identical. But absolutely identical? Probably not.

**Loss of sensation.** If you do lose nipple sensitivity after a reduction, most women regain sensitivity after a year or two. However, if you had a nipple transfer, that feeling will never return.

**Necrosis.** An ugly word for a horrific complication. It means dead tissue. In a reduction, where tissue is cut away and removed, the blood vessels need to pump oxygen to the area to heal the remaining tissue. If you have poor circulation, the oxygenated blood doesn't get to the area, and tissue doesn't heal. It can die, actually. And then you have a half-dead breast under your bra. The skin might turn black, and the breast might cave in around the dead tissue. It's a horrible result.

A major cause? Smoking! Smoking hinders circulation. When your doctor asks if you're a smoker, do not lie! When he tells you to quit for a month before surgery and two months after, do it or don't have the surgery.

## Breast Reconstruction

After a mastectomy, women can take heart in knowing their reconstruction will look gorgeous. Advances have been made in these surgeries, and new breasts are more natural-looking than ever before. There are two options for fashioning a new breast. The first is called "flap technique" and uses a woman's own body tissue. The second is using a tissue expander to stretch a woman's skin and then inserting a synthetic implant.

To construct a new breast mound using all natural materials, the surgeon will have to harvest donor muscle, fat, and skin from elsewhere on a woman's body and then move it to her chest. A "tram flap," aka "transverse rectus abdominis musculocutaneous flap," uses body tissue from the abdomen. A "latissimus dorsi flap" takes it from the back. An "S-gap flap" or "superior gluteal artery perforator flap" takes it from the butt.

With the tram and latissimus dorsi flaps, a surgeon can do a "pedicle flat" transfer, tunneling the donor skin/muscle to the chest without detaching it completely from its blood supply.

If he does have to do a "free flap" transfer, detaching the donor flap entirely, the relocated tissue will create new vessels to get a fresh supply of blood.

Once that surgery has healed—expect to have swelling, soreness, and bruising for up to six weeks in both the new breast and the donor area—the next (optional) step is nipple reconstruction. That procedure takes skin from another part of your body, the inner thigh, for example, and grafts it to the breast. The skin is tattooed for color. Just think of yourself as a younger Cher.*

"Flap technique breasts look natural," said Dr. Lisa Cassileth, a California surgeon who does a lot of breast reconstructions. "The problem is, you have to operate on two areas, so instead of a three-hour reconstruction with an implant, you have a five-hour surgery and a slower recovery."

The other technique, to reconstruct with an implant, is a longer process, if a shorter surgery. At the time of the mastectomy, the surgeon will put a tissue expander—a balloon with a valve—under the muscle of the chest wall. He can't just throw an implant in until the area is given a chance to expand. Every two weeks for several months, the surgeon will fill the tissue expander with more and more saline. When her skin is sufficiently stretched, the woman will have the expander taken out, and either a saline or silicone implant put in. This process takes longer, due to the gradual stretching of skin, but the implant surgery involves only one site and is shorter, easier, with a faster recovery. A nipple/areola reconstruction can be done after the implant surgery has healed, in about six weeks. A piece of skin is taken from a donor site, often the inner thigh, tattooed for color, and grafted onto the breast mound.

Any reconstruction after mastectomy will be covered by your medical insurance.

## Nipple Jobs

Bet you didn't even know that nipples had their own sub-specialty! Not many people do. Women who want to correct their nipples number in the thousands, and most of them do it in conjunction with another procedure like a lift or an augmentation. The vast majority

---

*Much* younger.

of nipple jobs are to correct inversion, where the nipple is tucked in on itself. Two percent of women have them—most were born that way—but some cases are due to internal scarring of milk ducts from breast-feeding.

Like breast ptosis, or degree of droop, there are levels of inversion in nipples. Grade 1, aka "shy nipples," are inverted but pop like turkey thermometers when treated with reverent kindness and/or touched. Grade 2: Deeper dents, which eventually will stick out, but only with a lot of effort. Grade 3: Severe indentation, like a mini-innie belly button on each boob, which never pop out, are useless for breast-feeding, get infected, and are prone to rashes.

## Reversion

To correct inverted nipples, of any grade, the surgeon will use a tiny scalpel and cut into the base of the nipple and lift it into a popped or protracted position. The fibers and ligature inside the nipple—which are too tight and cause the nipple to cave in—are then stretched and spread. The doctor takes care to make sure he doesn't damage milk ducts. Then he places some strategic stitches in the inside of the nipple and the base of it, to make sure the stretched fibers stay that way. For the next couple of days, you might have to wear a protective cup over your nipples to make sure they heal properly.

All told, it's a one-hour outpatient procedure, usually under local anesthesia, and costs only $1,000 to $4,000.

## Reduction

Nipple reduction—or making it shorter or narrower—is the easiest and simplest procedure in this chapter. To make them shorter, the doctor will, literally, take a little off the top. Just lop it right off and then suture or stitch it up. It'll heal in a few days and needs only an

"X" of Band-Aids across the boob.* The whole thing can be done with local anesthesia and costs only $1,000 to $3,000. To chip away at extra-wide nipples, the doctor will, likewise, give you a local anesthetic, and then cut away part of the nipple from the underside and then sew it up tight. It's like taking in, or putting darts in, a dress. Cost is in the $1,000 to $3,000 range.

Areola reduction is a bigger job and needs to be done under "light" general anesthesia. Even still, you can go home only a few hours after surgery. Like a doughnut incision breast lift (see page 154), the doctor will cut a circle around the areola at the circumference the patient desires. The excess-pigmented areola portion also gets a circular incision around it and is then removed. The remaining breast skin is connected to the smaller areola and sewn up. There are scars around the areola only. Cost: $2,000 to $5,000.

## Remind Me Again, Why Do I Want to Do This?

The rewards:

You can **breast-feed.** Women with grade-three inversions need surgery in order to nurse.

**Confidence.** You can **wear a white top.** Or a skimpy **bikini** or a crochet **bra.**

Your **boyfriend is safe** from impalement when he gets on top.

## What's the Worst That Could Happen?

The downsides:

**Complications.** Mainly, infection. But you'll probably be on a course of antibiotics before the surgery, so this is minimal. Infection is more likely to happen if the patient doesn't keep the incision wounds

---

*Pretend you're a contestant on "Hollywood Squares."

clean or doesn't wear the protective cups over the nipples for a few days or the post-op compression bra.

**Scars.** Only a danger in an areola reduction, really. You just never know how skin is going to heal, even if it's kept clean and your surgeon is a Michelangelo with a needle and suture. If you let the breast stretch (aka, if you don't wear a sports or compression bra post-op), your sutures might tug and that could mean weird scars around the areola like Tara Reid's trademark Bride of Frankenboob look. Minimize the risk by doing what your doctor tells you to do. Keep the wounds clean and bandaged, don't run a marathon the day after, etc.

**Sensitivity.** With boob jobs, the threat is loss of sensation. With nipple jobs? It's feeling way too much sensitivity. Your nipples will smart. They'll be pinpoints of ache for a day or two post-op. But when you heal, they'll feel normal.

## Celeb Boob Job Ticker

### In the "Now You See It, Now You Don't, Now You Do, Now You Don't Know What the Hell Is Going On" category:

**Pamela Anderson.** She changes her implants like other women change their mind. One marriage they're in, the next they're out, the next, they're in. It would be hard to keep abreast, if she weren't constantly posing nude. You could chart the stock market by Pam Anderson's cup size. Let's all hope she puts them back in and huger than ever.

**Jenna Jameson.** She had her first implants put in to once-and-for-all prove that big-chested blondes do well in the adult-film industry (you think?). She had those DDs taken out and had bigger ones put in. Maybe it was hard to see past (or over) her breasts. She eventually had the second implants removed and declared, optimistically, that her C-cups are half-full. Problem: her stretched-out skin makes them look half-empty.

## In the "Be Careful! Even the 'Best' Can End Up in Trouble" category:

**Courtney Love.** The widow/rock star/human experiment is famous for her shocking and outrageous behavior. Which I can appreciate. But no one wants shocking and outrageous boobs. Her implants are dented, cockeyed, and look like they're full of oatmeal.

**Vivica Fox.** In paparazzi photos, you can clearly see a deep dent on her right boob. Like it's a fender that got bendered. This is a case of stars with all the money in the world not choosing the right doctor or not following post-op instructions. Points off for the ding, but I do like her nose job.

**Tara Reid.** I pity this girl, with her oblong areolas, asymmetrical-sized and shaped boobs, and bad lipo scars. I'd feel better if she could keep them in her shirt! Which she can't.

## In the "More Is Less" category:

**Victoria Beckham.** She's achieved the long-coveted Tits on a Stick silhouette, although I wonder if she wanted to look like a pair of rock-hard soccer balls were shoved into her armpits.

**Janet Jackson.** If you're going to flash your breast for the entire world, it should look good! Her implants are so high and hard, they barely move when she dances. You can see her implant outline!

## In the "More Is More" category:

**Heidi Montag.** I've never watched her TV show "The Hills," but I like what I see of the hills on her chest. Her boosted boobs look natural and are in proportion with her body. Not too big, not too high. And she's public about doing it, which we like.

**Salma Hayek.** She says her boobs are real. The popular Hollywood opinion is that she's got implants, and they're so natural-looking, she can get away with her denials.

**Gisele Bündchen.** The underwear model reportedly went for medium instead of massive implants. The result? They give her curves where she needed them and made her the highest-paid model in the world.

( **Nine** )

# **Bobbing** for Noses

*Joan always had a big nose. The kind that would make Barbra Streisand stop and say, "Oy!" But even though Joan knew men adored women with perky, petite noses, she sniffed at the thought of getting hers fixed, opting instead for a less conventional way of minimizing the problem.*

*Joan's first day as curator of the Pinocchio Museum was everything she had hoped for, as neither tourist nor docent so much as glanced at her nose (now dwarfed by the super-sized schnozzes protruding from the faces of hundreds of wooden marionettes). Then an overnight termite infestation destroyed the entire puppet collection, leaving Joan a "sitting nose," so to speak, with nowhere to hide. All attention was focused again on Joan's protruding proboscis. As Japanese tourists clamored to pose for pictures with "The Rady Pinocchio," Joan decided to stop lying to herself and discreetly dialed a nose doctor to discuss her options. She then called Donna Karan, Céline Dion, Annie Leibovitz, and Barbra herself for moral support.*

• • •

Everyone knows the nose is the centerpiece of their face. It is literally front and center, an attention hog. And that's why Hollywood has had a long, strong tradition of stars getting rhinoplasty. Two hundred and eighty-five thousand people got a nose job in 2007, making it the third most popular plastic surgery of the year, right behind breast augmentation and liposuction.

Just about anything can be done (and has been) to the proboscis: a bump flattened, a tip tweaked, the nostrils narrowed, the sides slenderized. As Leonardo da Vinci explained to me once over Campari, "The nose sets the character for the whole face."

Sigmund Freud, that odd little Austrian, was as obsessed with the nose as he was with the penis. He had two operations on his own nose, both to fix the giant hole in his septum he got from snorting massive amounts of cocaine. Mucus ran from his nose continually. In his drug-induced haze, he likened it to vaginal fluid. Then, after observing that his lady patients reported nosebleeds during menstruation, he clapped his hands together and said, "Ah-ha! The nose is a tiny vagina." In one of his famous dreams, he examined the nasal cavity of Irma, a patient, and felt a strong desire to inject into it, with a "needle," the milky "solution" that she craved.

In Siggy's world, a nose wasn't always a nose.

As we've come to understand, Freud was a misogynist and a homophobe—as well as a downer at parties. Physiologically speaking, however, his theory of linking the nose and the vagina has some validity. The nasal septum is made of erectile tissue, like the clitoris and penis. As I've learned from my gentleman friends, Viagra makes their noses swell. Nosebleeds *are* common when women get their periods. Freud believed that, inside the nasal cavity, there are small spots that, when fingered, can turn you on.*

The first nose job in history was performed by a doctor named Sushruta in ancient India, circa 500 B.C. That's a 2,500-year-long tra-

---

*Before you go knuckle-deep hunting for the elusive N-Spot, trim your fingernails!

dition of nose fixing! Why does its shape and size matter so much? The small, pretty nose is a long-standing archetypal symbol of truth and goodness. We all know—and this is a proven fact—that when you lie, your nose grows and sprouts branches, complete with a bird's nest and eggs. The plucky down-on-her-luck princess always has a button nose. Her evil stepmother has a crooked, pointy, mangled, green-tinted snout. It's a hardwired-in-the-brain instinct to trust a balanced, well-proportioned face and associate it with honesty and loyalty. When a baby sees a face that's out of proportion—a nose that's too long or too wide—he'll cry. Shrinks have done studies.

Aristotle, the Greek father of philosophy, believed a hooked nose was a sign of intelligence. How did he reach this conclusion? He himself *had* a hooked nose. He was smart, ergo, ibid, ipso facto, *everyone* with a hooked nose was smart. Here's a theory of mine: men will twist any flaw to their own advantage. I bet Aristotle would've said a small penis was a sign of virility—if he had a small one, which I can't confirm.

I'm not *that* old.

Nose jobs are the ultimate balancing act of plastic surgery. A tiny tilt of the tip—which I had done—made a tremendous positive impact on my face. Do too much, and a woman can lose her unique character.

Jennifer Grey, star of *Dirty Dancing*, is an oft-cited example of a star whose dramatic nose job sandbagged her acting career. She used to have a distinctive nose, but her new bland one got Baby put in the corner for good.

There was a lot of chatter about Ashley Tisdale, a Disney star with a formerly distinctive nose, when she had her "deviated septum" fixed. (Funny and ironic, isn't it, that people so often lie about nose jobs, and, historically, lying is what makes the thing grow bigger!) Anyway, her quirky bump got chiseled away, and her look went from bold to blah. It's too early to tell if her new face will have her exiled from the Magic Kingdom.

Ann Miller, the dancing star of Hollywood's golden age, had her nose fixed, and it was way too small. Rumor had it that she had a prosthetic nose piece made for the movies. Her boyfriend, Louis B. Mayer, would take the piece with him when he went out of town so Ann couldn't leave the house.

Thank God the stigma about rhinoplasty is gone. People look at a teenage girl with a funny nose, and they ask, "Why *hasn't* she had that fixed?" Nose jobs are almost as standard as braces now. It's a rite of passage, and I'm all for it. Never mind throwing a big sweet sixteen party for your daughter. Put the money where it'll do lasting good: the best time to get your daughter's nose done is the summer before college. At a new school, she starts fresh. No one will register the change. They'll see only the beauty.

But, as with all plastic surgery, bad outcomes do happen when you tell the surgeon you want a certain star's nose. That celebrity might have a gorgeous one, but the shape of her nose might not look right on your face. Fortunately, most doctors have computer programs to show how different noses will look on you. I think there's a general perception that nose jobs are minor surgery, and that, since teenage girls get them, they aren't dangerous.

Wrong!

It's a big operation, under general anesthesia (usually). It's risky, and a bad nose job can ruin your looks, possibly, forever.

On the other hand, a good nose job can turn a *jolie laide* into Angelina Jolie.

A rhinoplasty requires tremendous surgical skill. For this procedure more than just about any other (except for face lifts), you must screen your doctor like your future happiness depends on it (FYI: it does). Pore over his before-and-after photos. Do you like what you see? Find out how many nose jobs he's done. There's an old expression that you have to hit 3,000 golf balls before you have a swing.

"Rhinoplasty is the most complicated and artistic of all plastic surgery," said Michigan-based surgeon Anthony Youn, M.D., author of the highly entertaining blog Celebrity Cosmetic Surgery (which mentioned me only twice). "Some surgeons with twenty years' experience say they feel like they're still only beginning to feel comfortable with rhinoplasty. I'd say a surgeon should have done fifty to one hundred in his lifetime. So he's not rusty, he should do a rhinoplasty at least every two weeks. Even then, some surgeons are only comfortable doing relatively simple operations, taking off a bump, for example. He'd have to be very experienced and brave to take on a complicated case, like Michael Jackson."

One more reason to count your blessings: you do not have Michael Jackson's nose. What's left of it.

## Small Parts

The nose is divided into twin chambers on either side of the septum. The septum is the wall of cartilage inside the nose (translucent white bendy matter; you've seen stuff like it many times when splitting chicken breasts). The septum serves both form (the tent pole that gives the nose shape and structure) and function (creating clear passageways for breathing). Remember the Hollywood scourge of the "deviated septum," the dread condition starlets like Ashlee Simpson, Jennifer Aniston, and Ashley Tisdale have suffered and had to have "corrected"? A deviated septum means you have holes in the cartilage (aggressive picking? Cocaine use? Afrin addiction?) or the septum has fallen to one side and can't get up (injury, bad genes). Aesthetics-wise, a deviated septum might mean a crooked nose, à la Owen Wilson. Health-wise, air passage could be blocked. What's a starlet to do? Nose job to the rescue. If she's not going to eat, at least she has to breathe! Might as well get her nose straightened, too.

Nostrils, we know all about. Nasal cavities are where the air goes in. The outward or lateral sides of the nose consist of cartilage (from the end to about halfway up) and bone (from the middle of the nose to where it meets the skull). The strip of skin between the nostrils that runs from the tip to where the nose meets your face is called the columella. Your nostrils are attached to the face by the alae.

Let's not forget the parts that give your nose "character," as da Vinci put it—the tip and the dorsal hump. The tip (aka, the greater alar cartilage) is the mass at the end of the nose. On the tip, you have the meaty substance called the alar fibro-fatty tissue. When a nose is called "bulbous," the bulb in question is ample alar tissue.

The dorsal hump is the bump on the bridge of the nose.

## To Shave a Dorsal Hump

Every year in the summer camp play, you were always cast as the witch. Or you've been described as having "strong" features or as a "handsome" woman. The hooked nose, otherwise known as "Roman" or aquiline, as well as the Grecian nose, a straight, strong line from forehead to nasal tip, might look good on "strong" and "handsome" men. On women? Of course, it's a matter of personal preference. Meryl Streep never had her dorsal hump shaved, yet her placement in the pantheon of "beauty" is secure.

But if you decide that the hump has got to go, you'll undergo either an "open rhinoplasty" or a "closed rhinoplasty."

An open rhinoplasty is what it sounds like. The skin of the nose is pulled back, so the doctor can operate on your open, exposed nasal bones and cartilage.

A closed rhinoplasty does not involve the removal of the skin on the nose. All the work is done through holes made in the nostril cartilage.

The closed technique was pretty much the gold standard until about twenty-five years ago when the open method became popular. Some doctors still prefer to do it the old-fashioned way, even though they're operating "blind." To shave a dorsal hump with a closed rhinoplasty, the doctor will cut holes in the nostril cartilage, into which he'll insert a tiny scalpel to shave away the excess cartilage on the septum. If need be, he'll insert a hammer into the holes to chisel away excess nasal bone by tapping the hammer with a mallet. He'll smooth down the chiseled bones with a "rasp," also inserted through the same holes. All excess cartilage and bone are removed with a forceps. A "closed" operation is fast, causes little bleeding, and the patient won't have any scars. Also, the patient can opt for local anesthesia. Your nose will be numb, but sorry, you'll be awake to the sounds and smells of your surgery.

Nowadays, most doctors use an open rhinoplasty to shave down a dorsal hump because they have better control over what they're doing. You'll have general anesthesia and be asleep for the length of the operation, some one to two hours—or possibly longer. The first step is to lift the nose skin. To do so, the doctor makes incisions inside your nostrils, at twelve o'clock, and a zigzag-shaped incision across the columella, the strip of skin between the nostrils. Next, he liberates the skin on your nose from the underlying cartilage and bone by cutting and pulling it back with a retractor. Your nose will be peeled like a grape. Your face will be normal, except for a skeleton nose in the middle. The process of pulling back the skin is called "skeletonizing"* the nose.

The bunched-up nasal skin is secured. On to getting rid of that dorsal hump. The surgeon has to remove excess cartilage on the septum and the lateral sides of the nose to give it a less Roman profile. To cut the soft cartilage, he'll use a scalpel. But when he gets to the bone on top, your doctor will use a chisel and a mallet to hammer away nasal bone. "The nasal bones aren't that hard," said Dr. Youn. "The other bones of the skull are much harder. In fact, when I'm working on a nose, I know I've gone too high when the bones become harder. To break the nasal bones, you only need to tap softly on the mallet. I like to make several small perforations, and then use my fingers to make the break." Like breaking a piece of matzoh? "Exactly. It can make a

---

*or Nicole Richie-izing

bone-crunching sound. This is one of the reasons I like general anes-thesia. The sound can upset the patient.*

Once the excess cartilage and bone that comprise the hump have been cut away, your surgeon will use a rasp—a surgical file—to soften the sharp edges of the newly chiseled bone. Then, since the cutting has left your nose de-roofed, your doctor will break the nasal bones on the sides, where they meet the face, and pinch them together over the septum to close the structure. (Incidentally, this is also how to thin a wide nose, with or without first shaving off a hump.)

Finally, the surgeon lowers the skin and sews the nostril carti-lage and the columella back together. He'll put some bandages on to minimize swelling and protect the fragile structure during the healing process. Post-op, you'll look like you've been hit in the face with a hammer. Maybe because you *have* been hit in the face with a hammer.

## To Shrink a Nasal Tip

If all your problems are to the point, meaning, on the tip of your nose, the doctor might not have to break bones! That's the good news. The bad news? He's still going to slice. Most tip-centric nose jobs are via the "open" method. It's easier to correct the bumps and bulges when they're exposed in their naked villainy. Once the doctor makes the appropriate cuts along the columella and inside the nostrils, he'll pull back the skin to expose the tip.

Grab the end of your nose and wiggle it around. The seemingly moveable bits are the alar cartilage and the alar tissue. Depending on what you need done, the doctor will use a scalpel to cut excess alar cartilage, thereby making the tip smaller, shorter, less pointy, what-ever you desire. I had my nose tip lifted, just turned up a bit, and it made a world of difference! In some cases, to narrow a too-wide tip,

---

*or Jews at Passover

the doctor will use sutures—surgical thread—to pull the two sides of the alar cartilage together. By sewing you up tight, he might not have to cut cartilage.

A word on cutting through cartilage: back to the raw chicken breasts we've all slapped around. When making, say, coq au vin, you use the whole breast sliced into manageable portions. To section a breast, one must cut through a band of cartilage—white, translucent, bendy matter. You can do so easily with a sharp knife. You could probably hack through it with a butter knife, but you'd mangle it in the process. On your nose, the surgeon will use a sharp scalpel and cut slowly and carefully.

I've seen pictures of bad cutting jobs: jagged, ripped cartilage. Not pretty.

"Even if you do cut cleanly, there's the potential problem of scar tissue formation," said Dr. Youn. "In order to heal, the nose forms scar tissue. Surgeons can't control how it grows. This is one reason to get rhinoplasty right the first time. With each successive surgery, you have more scar tissue and greater risk of not getting the outcome you want. Rhinoplasty is a surgery of millimeters. You can shave one millimeter off the tip, for example, and two millimeters of scar tissue might form. I tell patients, each time they have their nose done their expectations have to decrease."

Sarah Jessica Parker has, allegedly, had her formerly rather large tip tweaked in as many as three different nose jobs. She must have a lot of scar tissue, because her nose shape is still not small. But as they say, "She looks a lot better." Besides, a too-cute nose on her face could have doomed her to Jennifer Grey-ville.

## Narrower

When Beyoncé allegedly got her nose slenderized, she probably had her lateral (side) nasal bones broken and pushed inward to bring the bridge of her nose to a more defined point. This can be done without having to cut cartilage (as with shaving a dorsal hump). Beyoncé might also have had a certain procedure to narrow wide-set nostrils, too. It's called a Weir excision. The surgeon makes snips at the nasal base (not to be confused with a naval base), where the outside of the nostril connects with your face. He removes a bit of extra flesh and then stitches what's left together, narrowing the nostril opening. Imagine a circle (the nostril opening). Cut part of the circle away, and then re-close the ends. What do you get? Smaller circle.

The scars are small and hidden in a natural crease. Undetectable. If you also have an extra-long nasal tip shortened, you'll need a Weir excision, too, to prevent a bunch-up of extra skin.

## Shorter

Go find a mathematical compass. I suggest checking your kid's backpack or an old desk. You can also find one in any antique shop, right next to that genuine Louis XIV iPod.

Got it? Now measure the angle created between the upper lip and the columella—the strip of skin between the nostril openings. This is called the nasolabial angle. The perfect nasolabial angle, for men, is 90 degrees. For the ladies, it's 100 degrees. If your nose is long and bends downward, the nasolabial angle is too small and your nose is too long. The only good thing with this is you can stop and smell the flowers without having to bend over.

Your surgeon has many options here, including nipping the tip and shortening the septum/lateral nasal cartilage in an open rhinoplasty.

## Straighter

Paging Cameron Diaz! Reportedly, the blond actress's nose was broken a few times over the course of her young life, which gave her a deviated septum (!), which caused breathing problems. Cameron

Diaz, snorer? Too sad and tragic. She got a nose job to have her right-leaning septum pushed back to the center of her face. Good for her. She had a crooked nose, and now it looks nicer. Why couldn't she just say she didn't like how it looked and wanted it fixed? Why insist that she had it done *only* for health reasons? Why not say, "I was getting the septum fixed, so I had them straighten me out, too."

If you have a crooked nose, then you most likely have a bent septum. The procedure to straighten it out is called a septoplasty. Using an open or closed rhinoplasty, the doctor will cut away the part of the septum that's bending into one of your nasal cavities and blocking airflow. If a lot of septum is removed, the doctor might harvest extra cartilage from your ear or another part. In some cases, you'll have little baby-sized splints inserted to support your new septum. They'll come out a week or so after the surgery. Through the nostrils.

"Several months after surgery, straightened cartilage might warp and change shape," said Dr. Youn. Even if your nose looks perfect a month later, it can always bend again, from warping or the buildup of scar tissue.

## Larger

A nose that's too delicate for your face can be pumped up. Only way to do it, obviously, is to add to what's already there, and that means implants. Little silicone implants can work well. "In Asian cultures, to make noses more Caucasian-looking, they use an L-shaped implant,* from the root of the nose between the eyes to the tip," said Dr. Youn.

It's preferable to use cartilage from the patient's own body. If someone else's cartilage is used, the body will reject it coldly. Your nose welcomes with open nostrils the cartilage from your own ear or bone from your rib, which the surgeon will graft onto your current structure, like adding a sun room to your house.

*Or R-shaped, as it's known in China.

# Tweaking

Say, back in the seventies, you got a nose job in the then-trendy "ski-jump" style, and now you want more volume along the bridge of the nose. A procedure that's gaining in popularity is using fillers, in this case, Restylane, to add volume to the nose. It's a valid non-invasive procedure for someone who doesn't want surgery. People think of it as a lunchtime nose job: get a shot of filler for a minor touch-up or to fix a small defect.

But it isn't risk-free. You might have lumpiness, unevenness, tissue rejection of the filler. It's temporary, too. At some point, getting Restylane shots in the nose every six months might not be cost-effective. If you do the math, it might be worth it to get the permanent solution of rhinoplasty.

# Not Gonna Happen

You can't change the snout of a pig into the beak of a sparrow, no matter how much money you spend. Have a frank talk with your doctor about what he can and can't do.

Remember, a plastic surgeon's favorite words are "realistic" and "expectations."

## What's This Gonna Cost Me?

According to the American Society of Plastic Surgeons, the national average fee for a rhinoplasty is $4,000. But since each nose is unique, with its own humps and hooks, you can pay less, or a lot more, up to $7,500, depending on your nose needs. A closed rhinoplasty to simply narrow a wide nose would be less expensive than an open rhinoplasty with a tip reduction, dorsal hump removal, and re-roofing. Basically, if you need to fix a nose like Barry Manilow's—the man who from New York can smell the smog in Los Angeles—you'll be on the high end of the range.

## Remind Me Again, Why Do I Want to Do This?

The rewards:

**No one will ever call you Hawk Face again.** I say this for the teenage girls who dream of a cuter nose. Kids can be cruel. We all want to fit in with the community of our peers, while standing out for our individuality. No one wants to stand out for having a beak.

Parents: When your kid hits sixteen—the youngest age doctors will perform a rhinoplasty—let her (or him) have the nose job she's been begging for. It's an act of kindness, which she'll appreciate for the rest of her life.

**You have eyes now.** The thing about a prominent nose: It's an attention hog. It's the first thing you look at in the mirror. It's the first part of you to enter a room. In conversation, no one makes eye contact with you because they're staring at your nose. Once you've been fixed, suddenly mascara, liner, and shadow have a purpose! People will start to say things like, "Have you always had such beautiful blue eyes?"

**Photos of you from more than one angle.** People who've had a lifetime of being self-conscious about their noses have figured out their best angle and presented it for the camera compulsively. Grab a stack of old pix. There's you, three-quarter view, in front of the Grand Canyon. There's you, three-quarter view, in front of the Eiffel Tower. Well, now you can pose with your profile in front of the Statue of Liberty.

**Confidence! Self-Esteem! Win by a nose!** Having a nose job is like getting over a hump, literally and figuratively. Once you've gotten rid of what's been holding you back, the rush of confidence will astonish you. Look what it does for women who divorce their deadbeat husbands.

## What's the Worst That Could Happen?

The risks:

**Death.** I always start big and go down from there. Any time you have general anesthesia, there is a chance something could go wrong, and you won't wake up. I don't like to say it; I have to.

**Complications.** Bleeding through the N-holes. If this happens, you'll get civilized packing from your doctor until the leaky vessels heal. You might get an infection, also, but probably not if your doctor gives you pre-operative antibiotics.

**Scarring.** *Rarely* are the columella and Weir excision scars more noticeable than you might like. Although you won't enjoy it, your doctor can cut away bad scars and try again to stitch seamlessly.

**Pain.** Degree of "discomfort?" High. Remember what I said about being hit in the face with a hammer? Nose jobs are uncomfortable. You can be relieved of the worst of it with painkillers. They'll keep you numb and relaxed for the first few days. Most likely, your nose will be stuffed like a turkey with gauze.

Fortunately, it'll be immediately relieved the blessed moment the packing comes out a few days later. Give it two or three weeks before all tenderness and twinges go away.

**Swelling.** You've just spent $5,000 for a smaller nose. You look in the mirror, post-op, and your nose appears to have been inflated with helium. It could be a float in the Macy's Thanksgiving Day parade, right behind the one of my thighs. Swelling is part of recovery. Fortunately, it'll go down and quickly. By the end of the first week—if you're vigilant with the ice pack—you'll have a pretty good idea of what your new nose looks like. By the end of the month, eighty percent of the swelling is gone. You'll have to wait six months, though, to see your new nose in a pristine state of healing.

**Bruising.** Expect shiners—Rocky Balbo–style. Big black-and-blue beauties under your eyes. Go outside before the week's out, and your neighbor might call a domestic violence hotline on your behalf. Until the bruising disappears in a couple of weeks, makeup helps.

**Disappointment.** Have I mentioned that disappointment is a severely underestimated emotion? Never more so than fantasizing for decades about a new nose, only to look in the mirror and think, "Eh." Or worse, "Feh." I won't lie to you. Rhinoplasty has a high rate of repeat surgeries. There's cartilage warping to worry about. And scar tissue formation.

## Worst Nose Job Ever Department
*Michael Jackson*

The two scariest words associated with plastic surgery and children's playgrounds. It's a national tragedy, how such a talented young pervert transformed himself into a freak of suture. Only in America would a black man turn himself into a white woman. Forget the wigs, bleached skin, chin dimple, cheek implants, chin implant, and tattooed eyeliner. Let's concentrate on Michael's nose, or lack thereof. What the hell *happened?*

"Stating the obvious, he's had too many nose jobs," said Dr. Youn. "Each reduction rhinoplasty removed more cartilage to make his nose smaller and thinner. Cartilage is what gives the nose a shape. Jackson's has been whittled down to the point that there's nothing left to support it. In the place of cartilage, he's got massive amounts of scar tissue, which is why Jackson's nose appears jagged, gnarled, and dented. He probably has a saddle-nose deformity—when the nose has a big dent on the bridge that looks like a saddle—among many other problems. I heard at one point that he had a silicone implant put in to support his nose, but that his body rejected it and was pushing it out. When he was on trial for child molestation and appeared in court with bandages all over his face, the chatter was that his implant was being forced out through a hole in his skin."

Regarding the skin on top of Jackson's nose, Dr. Youn added, "It's thinned beyond repair. Whenever you lift the skin off a nose to do a rhinoplasty, the skin thins and forms a small amount of scar tissue. If it weren't for the scar tissue, he'd probably have nothing holding the skin together."

Is there no hope for Jackson's thin-skinned, scarred-up little mess? "The only way to re-create his nose is to treat it as a cancer reconstruction," said Dr. Youn. "He'd have to have the skin on his forehead rotated down to cover his nose, or that contracted knob of scar tissue he's got for a nose. The procedure is called a para medial forehead flap. He'd also need some bone grafting, taking bone from his ribs, to give the nose shape."

Suffice it to say, a forehead flap isn't a quick and easy lark of a surgery. An upside-down nose-shaped patch of skin is cut into the forehead and then swung down to cover the nose. The skin on our forehead, minus the nose-shaped cutout, is sewn together on either side of the incision. If Jackson had this done, he'd have significant scars down the middle of his forehead, across the bridge of the nose, along the lateral sides of the nose, and around the tip.

As Dr. Youn joked, Jackson would be no "pretty young thing," as his famous song goes.

Anything would be an improvement!

# Celeb Nose Jobs Ticker

## In the "Less Is More" category:

**Marilyn Monroe:** A little thinning changed her from a pretty farm girl into the World's Sexiest Woman.

**Beyoncé:** A slight narrowing took her from pretty to booty-licious.

**Winona Ryder:** By thinning her tip, she looked more feminine, delicate, and sexy. A small change for dramatic effect.*

## In the "More Is More" category:

**Cher:** Does anyone remember her nose from "The Sonny and Cher Show"? It was big and made her look cross-eyed. A total revamp turned her into a goddess.

## In the "Did She, or Didn't She?" category:

**Gwyneth Paltrow:** Her alleged reduction made her new nose fit with her fine features. Now if they could just do the same with her gigantic ego.

**Angelina Jolie:** Her puffy nose allegedly narrowed, Mrs. Brad Pitt went from weird to wow.

**Katie Holmes:** An apparent tiny slenderizing of the nose, rumored to be via rhinoplasty, gave her a more mature look. Or maybe she's aged years since becoming a Stepford Wife.

## In the "Less Is Less" category:

**Jennifer Grey:** Who knew that her nose was her mojo? After she got it fixed, Baby got fewer parts.

**Ashlee Simpson:** She lost the bump and her "edge."

**Tori Spelling:** Her nose is mangled with scar tissue and just looks bad.†

---

*Plus store security cameras no longer recognize her when she shoplifts.
†See what happens when you're cut out of the will, Melissa?

**Courtney Love:** Train wreck. And it collided with the middle of her face.

## Deviated Septum Victims:

**Jennifer Aniston:** A nose job denier until she was forced to admit to it. And then she used the deviated septum line. It's like pleading the Fifth!

**Ashley Tisdale:** Thanks to her "deviated septum" surgery, she's gone from bold to blah.

**Cameron Diaz:** She got her crooked septum straightened and looks better than ever.

# ( Ten )

# Sucks to Be You: Lipo!

*Joan hated the fat pockets above her knees but refused to consider liposuction as an option. As summer began, she needed to find new and creative ways to conceal them. Kneepads were certainly a solution, but she didn't want people to mistake her for Monica Lewinsky. She considered strapping herself to a skateboard and panhandling outside the bus station, but she knew she could never be mistaken as a Vietnam vet, and they were the only ones who made good money. If only Joan had had ties to the underworld, she could have hired a thug to whack her in the knees with a baseball bat so she'd have an excuse to keep them covered.*

*Joan finally settled on a less painful solution—attending a dance class where she could meet single (and hopefully straight) men while keeping her knees covered doing the Charleston. It worked! Joan hit it off with a fellow dance student who was also a Broadway talent agent. He arranged for her to audition for the show Chicago. Joan did wonderfully until she was asked to sing "All That Jazz" and throw her leg up on a chair, revealing her grotesquely fat knee. She was stopped abruptly by the director, who told her that he saw talent and that she was an attractive girl (the other work was really paying off), but with knees like that, there was only one place for her on Broadway—as the lead in the* Teletubbies On Ice *show. That very afternoon, Joan phoned a liposuction doctor and went to see him during the first rehearsal break.*

Americans love skinniness, but we're the fattest country in the world. Call it the American paradox. We just can't pull our faces out of the feed bag!

Personally, I love food. When they throw rice at a wedding, I eat it.

Like Paris Hilton, I'll put anything in my mouth.

My picture of praying hands has a sandwich in it.

I go to KFC and lick everyone else's fingers.

But I know when I have to scale back. It's time to start a diet when the DMV says I've got to wear headlights. Or when I go to the beach, and the whales watch *me*.

I try to eat right, but finding time for fruits and vegetables on a daily basis is a challenge. (It's not enough that I visit my gay Uncle Leo and comatose cousin, Nadia, every two months.)

Ultimately, diets never work. The only woman who ever lost ten pounds and kept them off was Marie Antoinette.

And diet aids? They're all bull. Have you heard of the miracle diet pill Hoodia? More like Hoodwinkia.

Even if I could reach my ideal weight, pockets of flab would stick to my ass like superglue. You might be in decent shape and still have flabby upper arms or hate handles (only optimists call them "love handles"). Even marathon runners and anorexics have fat deposits. If you want to blame someone, point the finger of blame at the two people you blame for your divorce, smoking, drinking, bad dreams, and bedwetting. That's right. I'm talking about Mother and Father. Your parents gave you the genes that make you spill over your jeans like a muffin top. Diets fail because your body size and the way you gain weight are all genetic. I got my eyes from Mom, my nose from Dad, and my hips from the Cossack my Grandma schtupped back in Minsk.

Genetics dictate where you store extra fat and how you burn it off. Conventional wisdom dictates that the first place you gain weight is the last place you'll lose it. For example, you'll get skinny in your elbow before you shed an ounce from your ass. Even if you don't, your genes know your ass from your elbow. And your genetic predisposition will have you sitting on that cushion forever.

No wonder they call it the bitter end.

My theory—and this is backed up by personal trainers from Bel Air to Bangkok—is that no one loses stubborn fat pockets (saddlebags or stomach pouches) through dieting because they quit in frustration long before they make a dent.

Don't you love that phrase: "stubborn fat"? It's like the fat refuses to ask for directions when it gets lost.

I can name a dozen women—slim by any standard—who have been consumed with self-hatred over small pockets of fat. Which brings us to liposuction. Three hundred and two thousand people had their fat sucked out in 2007, making it the year's second most popular cosmetic surgery!

## Suck You?

Liposuction—literally, vacuuming the fat from your bulges—can be done to a substantial area, like your saddlebags, or a small one, like your neck. You can suck out as little as a syringe of schmaltz from your chin waddle or a gallon of gunk from your rear end. Liposuction can be done in many, many places. Around the ankles. The armpit/bra bulge. Above the knees. The upper arms. Love handles. The spare tire. I could go on. And on. The point: lipo is great for slimming the pockets, but it's useless for the whole suit. That's why doctors call it "body contouring," instead of "body minimizing." Liposuction is not a diet. It's not a weight-loss program. You have to be in fairly decent shape to get hoovered.

Ergo, if you're obese, I'm sorry, but it's not the answer. Reputable doctors won't come near you with a ten-foot suction pump. Don't be fooled by urban legends of women having fifty pounds of fat aspirated (sucked out) in a single day. My doctor friends laughed in my face when I asked if that were feasible. Maybe it was attempted in the olden days of lipo, when it first became popular in the 1980s. But those stories had tragic endings. People died after high-volume lipo from blood loss, embolisms, shock.

These days, the only shocking thing about lipo is the price (more on that later). People rarely, if ever, die via lipo anymore. It's considered one of the safest techniques around—because doctors know their limits. The maximum amount of fat that can be safely sucked out on any given day on any given person is 5,000 ccs, roughly eleven pounds (aka the Olsen twins' combined weight). Any more puts your health at risk. If you weigh 400 pounds, you'd need to have lipo twenty-five times over a period of years, spending hundreds of thousands of dollars, to be a normal weight.

Instead, you could try the Joan Rivers Diet. It works for me. Whenever I look in the mirror, I throw up.

## Know Your Enemy

Fat. You know what kills me? When people say, "You can lose fifty pounds of ugly fat!" What I want to know is, who the hell ever saw fifty pounds of *pretty* fat? You've been acquainted with fat your whole life. Happily, now you can get rid of some of it, in some areas, under the right conditions.

Fat basics: you are born with billions of fat cells. Unless you become morbidly obese, the fat cells you're born with are all you're ever going to have. The cells don't multiply, but they do get bigger and smaller as you gain and lose weight. You can't lose a cell completely, unless you have it sucked out of your body via liposuction. A fat cell can't be destroyed, unless the membrane is ruptured by ultrasonic high-frequency radio waves or zapped with a laser. (The future of flab—available today! Details to come.) If you sucked out fat cells via liposuction, fat will never again accumulate in that area. Which reminds me of another urban legend about the woman who had full body liposuction and then gained sixty pounds in her neck.*

We think of fat as the horrible layer that comes between us and a six-pack. Actually, the six-pack of beer is what comes between you and a waistline. You have an epidermis (outer layer of skin, what we can see on ourselves in private and on Lindsay Lohan in public). Under that, we have the dermis, deep layers of skin. Under that, we have a fat layer. Under that, the well-cushioned muscles. Fat can be found protecting some tissue and organs, like the stomach and intestines, in a good way. Fat can also be found clogging some tissue and organs, like the blood, liver, and heart, in a bad way.

You hate fat, but it's not really your enemy. We need stores of it for energy, insulation, to maintain body temperature, and enjoy proper body function. Essential vitamins A, D, E, and K are fat-soluble, meaning they are absorbed and digested via fat. Without fat in your diet, your hair and nails would be brittle and dry. A woman with extremely low body fat (less than 20 percent)—marathoners, anorexics—lacks the energy stores to support a fetus† and becomes infertile. If you had zero fat in your diet, you wouldn't be able to digest food.

But, for all the good it does, there's still no earthly reason you need it wobbling around under your chin.

---

*This would have been a life-saver for Marie Antoinette.
†Reminds me of when Nicole Richie was pregnant and anorexic. She was eating for one.

# A Slurpy History: The Early Years of Liposuction

Scientists split the atom seventy years ago. They put a man on the moon half a century ago. You'd think sucking the fat out of a stomach bulge through a tube would've been perfected by medieval surgeons in deerskin aprons. In fact, liposuction, or lipoplasty as we know it, is only 35 years old.

I've got hemorrhoids older than that.

Liposuction was born in Italy, improved in France, refined in America, advanced in Colombia, and, closing the loop, perfected back in Italy.

You can trace its blubbery trail across three continents.

In 1974, Italian gynecologist Dr. Giorgio Fischer looked up from his frittata and cappuccino one morning, turned to his gynecologist son, Dr. Giorgio Jr., and said, *"Ciao!* What would happen if we stuck a small, electrically powered rotating scalpel inside the flabby belly of a woman and vacuumed out her fat through a hose?" What happened wasn't pretty. Early patients—guinea pigs—suffered hemorrhages, permanent numbness, shock, deformities, nerve damage, tissue damage, blood vessel damage. The ones who lived didn't care: they were thin!

Next stop, France, the country where women don't get fat. Well, apparently, they do. Otherwise, French plastic surgeon Dr. Yves-Gerard Illouz wouldn't have had live patients to practice on. Over a breakfast of croissants and café au lait in 1977, he said to himself, *"Alors!* If I used a flat, blunt-edged cannula instead of a rotating blade, maybe the lipo patients wouldn't need emergency blood transfusions or go into shock." Indeed, using the cannula—a steel tube—maimed or injured far fewer patients than the Italian flying scalpels. Progress! Using the cannula to tunnel into the fat layer became the standard approach. In collaboration with another French doc, Dr. Pierre-François Fournier, Illouz improved the technique further by first infusing the area to be sucked with saline, epinephrine (a hormone that tightens blood vessels), and lidocaine (a pain killer). Patients bled less, but lipo still left them battered and bumpy.

Enter California dermatologist Dr. Jeffrey Klein. In 1985, over a breakfast of granola and carrot juice, he wondered, "What if I *flooded* the area with fluid, using two or three times as much of the saline/epinephrine/lidocaine solution as those Frenchies?" Klein, thusly, invented what we now call "tumescent liposuction." By pumping three times as much solution into the area as the amount of fat he intended to remove, the fat came out easier, thereby protecting nerves, tissues, and vessels.

## Tumescent Lipo at a Glance

Tumescent lipo is now the standard operating procedure. Depending on where you have it done, specifics vary, of course: incision location, quantity of fat removed, and duration of the treatment. Regardless of the area, however, the basic progression of steps is the same:

As with most operations, you'll get an IV drip of antibiotic beforehand. Then you'll pose nude (hussy!) while your doctor draws a road map on your body of where he'll remove fat. You'll submit to the body art standing up. Since you'll be walking around in your bikini, not lying flat on your back, the guidelines are made with you upright. Some doctors do lipo on an operating table that rotates into a nearly vertical position, making it even clearer how to contour the fat for a biped humanoid.

After you're been marked, you'll lie down on the table (or sit up in the chair for, say, neck lipo). If you're getting general anesthesia, good night. We'll talk again in a few hours. Those of you on the local anesthesia, you'll now be served your sedative. The lipo area will then be injected with a numbing agent.

When you can feel no pain, the doctor will make the incision in the skin to insert a cannula into the fat layer between the dermis and the muscle wall. A cannula, you remember, is a long tube with perforations, or small holes, on the end. The first cannula is hooked up to a machine that pumps a liquid solution of lidocaine (painkiller), epinephrine (to contract blood vessels), and saline into your body. The lipo area will be infused with the solution while the doctor massages the area, pumping the cannula to dowse into all the right places and to loosen the fat.

The next step is to insert the aspiratory cannula. This one is hooked up to a suction machine. The cannula is also connected to a tube through which your fat will travel to its final destination and plastic measuring vessels which look like kitchenware. While the fat is being vacuumed out, if you're awake, you will feel movement and pressure. If you're positioned fortuitously, you'll be able to watch the fat and solution move through the tubing into the vessels.

You probably assume the fat is yellow and gunky, like chicken fat. It would be, except the saline solution makes it pink and slushy like a drink from 7-Eleven. While all this sucking is going on, your doctor will be contouring the area. He'll make sure the remaining fat (some has to be left behind as a necessary cushion between the skin and the underlying muscle and organs) is uniform.

Next, you'll be cleaned and stitched up (if necessary—many incisions are so small, you won't need sutures). Doctors are very good about finding the natural crease or discreet spot for the incisions. Arm lipo incisions are usually placed, artfully, in the armpit crease. Neck lipo incisions are neatly tucked under the chin or by the ears. The tummy lipo entry point and exit point is often inside the belly button. Butt lipo marks are along the crease where butt meets thigh. That way, the stitches and scars will be hidden.

You'll be fit into a compression garment to prevent swelling. The garment is key for contouring. "You selectively contour the fat, leaving a layer beneath the skin. The greatest amount is removed in the area of maximum bulging and with decreasing amounts removed approaching the areas of normal contour," said Scott Zevon, M.D., fellow of the American College of Surgeons, board certified by the American Board of Plastic Surgery, a clinical instructor of plastic surgery at Columbia University College of Physicians and Surgeons, and one of *New York* magazine's best plastic surgeons in NYC. "After the surgery, wearing a compression garment helps resolution of swelling and may facilitate the treated final contour."

General anesthesia patients will spend the night or stay in the recovery room for several hours. All lipo patients can walk and move around, if gingerly, after surgery.

## Melting Innovations

After the tumescent revolution, doctors continued to invent new techniques to increase safety, minimize pain and bleeding, and speed recovery time. Not all of their innovations have been successful.

Dr. Michele Zocchi, another Italian, came up with the idea of holding paddles just above the skin that emit ultrasonic waves prior to suctioning the fat. The high-frequency sound waves pulsed through the outer layer of skin, reached the layer of fat cells, and heated up the cells, causing their membranes to burst and the fat inside the cells to liquefy. Hot, emulsified, free-flowing fat was easier to suck out than cold, hard globs. Two big problems with so-called external ultrasound-assisted lipoplasty: 1) the paddles burned patients' skin, and 2) docs had a hard time contouring the lipo'ed area.

You wanted a tight, flat belly, but you walked away with bad burns and lumps. The downsides were too extreme, and the technology became obsolete.

"Companies are working on new external ultrasound machines with improved technology, as compared to the existing machines," said Dr. Zevon. "They will likely be for smaller-volume fat deposits. We'll see how they do when they become available."

Internal ultrasound liposuction applies the same ideas as used today to great success and fewer side effects. After a tumescent solution is inserted via a cannula, the Vaser probe goes in, emitting high-frequency sound waves that heat and break up fat cells. "I use a Vaser," said Dr. Cassileth. "It's for fibrous fat on the back, upper abdomen, and for men who are having a gynecomastia, or breast reduction procedure."

Next big idea: putting a motor on the cannula so the doctor doesn't have to break a sweat pumping it back and forth himself. You've probably seen lipoplasty on TV or in movies. It looks like the doctor is stabbing someone in the gut, or wherever, with the cannula. The stabbing motion is actually the process of tunneling through dense, thick fat to loosen and remove it. The motorized cannula speeds up and eases fat removal as well as allows the doctor to concentrate on contouring and not burning his bicep muscles. This is called "power-assisted lipoplasty," and it's widely used today.

The real giant leaps forward in lipo technology have taken place in the last ten years. Colombian surgeon Dr. Rodrigo Neira came up with a new way to melt fat before it gets sucked out. He invented a laser device to hold over the body, like the ultrasonic paddles. What's different about the laser: the light waves are cold. No more burns. Also, the laser targets *only* fat cells. No blood vessels or tissues are damaged. The laser-melted fat is oily and easy to suck out or to just drain out through a tube.

Sometimes, suction and drainage aren't necessary at all. The small but significant amount of liquefied fat—50 ccs, a bit less than two ounces—from your neck, say, or knee, can be absorbed by your body.

## Genius of Lipo

The latest, greatest, giant leap for liposuction, developed in Italy, is the lipolysis technique, using a fiber-optic laser inserted into the body to liquefy fat before sucking it out. It's been done in South America and Europe for nearly a decade. The Smartlipo™ lipolysis machine won FDA approval in 2007. It's legal, if not readily available, since most doctors don't have one yet.*

The technique uses a hair-thin cannula with a laser on the tip. The cannula is inserted into the fat pocket. In a dark room, you can see the pinpoint of laser light underneath your skin. Using a back and forth motion, the doctor pumps the cannula, melting fat with the laser. As he goes, the area changes from hard fat to soft mush. Since the cannula is so thin, you won't need stitches to close the tiny incision holes.

Next, fat removal. Because the fat has been melted, the aspiration cannula can be super-thin, like a strand of angel-hair pasta. The fat is the consistency of olive oil, and it slides though the micro-cannula easily. Micro-cannula equals mini-scars, if any. Less blood loss, less trauma. Quicker healing. The recovery period is a third as long as traditional tumescent lipo.

Also, since Smartlipo is done under local anesthesia, it's cheaper, too, so you'll be able to afford a plate of angel-hair pasta with olive oil to celebrate.

## What's This Gonna Cost Me?

The cost depends on where you get sucked, how much you have sucked, and whether you're awake or asleep during the procedure.

*I'm buying my plastic surgeon one for Christmas.

If you have, say, the maximum amount of 5,000 ccs removed from the mid-section (a tricky operation—the doctor has to break up hard pack from the belly, hate handles, and back bacon while avoiding the nearby vital organs), it will cost you from $5,000 to $10,000. Throw in a tummy tuck to tighten up loose skin around your vacuumed middle, add a few thousand, plus the cost of general anesthesia. The operation could last up to five hours. Total cost range: $8,000 to $13,000.

Now, say you're looking to eliminate a mere 100 ccs from your neck. You'll do it under local anesthesia, meaning you'll be comfortably numb yet awake (and, thank God, sedated, too). The operation will only last an hour, and you'll walk out of the office on your own feet, holding your newly thinner chin high, or as high as you can in the mummy-like compression headpiece. Cost of lipo-lite: $2,500 to $5,000.

## Remind Me Again, Why Do I Want to Do This?

The rewards:

**A friendly mirror.** Before, when you looked in the mirror, your eyes went immediately to the precise spot of your disdain. The bulge, the pouch, the jiggle. You were flooded with frustration and/or self-loathing. Well, liposuction not only removes the fat from your trouble area, it sucks out your self-loathing, too. When you look in the mirror post-lipo, your eyes will go immediately to what used to give you heartburn, but now fills your heart with pride and joy. Self-loathing turns into self-love. "I'm hot," you think. "I'm a rock star. I go, girl."

**Jeans fit!** Farewell, muffin-topping.

**Bikinis are doable!** Picture you, jogging down the beach in a red bikini, your flat stomach and visible abs gleaming in the sun.

**Visible jawline!** You have a profile again.

It all adds up to **confidence, relief** and **gratitude**, which we can all use more of.

**Turn that point.** A lot of doctors report that lipo is a turning point for patients. The fat was a hurdle they couldn't get over. But once it was gone, they were able to change their lifestyles, make healthy choices, start working out, eat better, and think happy thoughts about their bodies. Women lose weight—and keep it off. Lipo shouldn't be seen as a weight-loss method before you have it, but it's a great motivator afterward.

## What's the Worst That Can Happen?

The risks:

**Death.** As always, I have to include the worst-case scenario. People do die of lidocaine toxicity, fluid overload, blood loss, blood clots, fat in the lung. If you use a board-certified doctor and have the procedure done at an accredited facility, your chances of dying are slim to none.

**Infection.** Always a danger when you're cut. Usually, the doctor will have you on antibiotics before and after, so the risk is small.

**Tissue damage.** Doctors, regardless of what their mothers say, are human.* They can make a mistake, slip up a bit, and jam the cannula into a vital organ. No one wants a holey lung or a punctured bowel. It's rare. Hardly EVER happens with a good doc.

**Blood loss.** You will lose some blood, but not nearly as much as patients used to in the pre-tumescent days. If you lose too much, you'll get a transfusion. It's not a bad idea to put some of your own blood aside in case a transfusion becomes necessary.

**Bruising.** You will have bruises. Temporarily! They'll look better in two weeks.

**Swelling.** You will swell. Temporarily! It'll go down progressively, up to six months. After only six weeks, 80 percent of the swelling will

---

*Except for Josef Mengele.

be gone. Wearing a compression garment over the area for four weeks helps a lot with girth control and smoothing the new surface of your fat-free skin.

**Pain.** You will have some pain. But you will also have drugs to help you forget about it. After a week, you can go back to work, housewifery, or your ordinary lady-of-leisure activities.

**Lumps.** Remember the anatomy. If you remove a fat cell, it's gone forever. Nothing will take its place. Therefore, if your doctor isn't careful about contouring, and if you don't wear your compression garment for the full four to six weeks, you might find lumps, an uneven surface, asymmetry, or dents in the area.

**Sagging skin.** If you're having a lot of fat removed, and your skin isn't as springy as it used to be, you might wind up with folds and sags that are just as unsightly as the bumps and bulges. You might not know beforehand how well your skin will contract after, so it's hard to predict if you'll need tightening until six months down the road. You can have the skin lifted, of course. But it's another operation.

**Scarring.** With the newfangled micro-cannulas, scars are getting smaller and smaller, and they're well hidden. Depending on where your incision was made, you might not even notice your scar. But, the real possibility is that you will. A famous starlet had stomach lipo, and the incision scars, dotted all over her belly like Morse Code, are plainly visible in bikini paparazzi shots. That's a sign of bad placement more than anything. If you're freaked out by scars, talk to your doctor about incision placement. Scars do fade over time. And tiny ones can always be written off as love bites.

**Disappointment.** Women get lipo and expect to wear size two jeans the next day. Six months is a long time to wait for the swelling to go down. And even then, you might have lumps, scars, or loose skin to deal with. Women who dreamed of a flat tummy will be saddened that, although a lot of flab was removed, the intra-abdominal fat (the material marbled throughout your organs that can only be dieted away) was left behind. If you've got a lot of it, your belly will continue to bulge.

**Regaining the weight.** Perhaps the worst thing about the post-lipo-life is the threat of regain. Since your fat cells were removed permanently—and you can never gain weight in those places—if you pack on pounds after the operation, it might look weird. Lumpy, asymmetrical, in puffy lines and patterns, divots or dents. If you'd never had lipo and gained weight, you'd look fatter. If you had lipo and you gain weight, you'll look bizarre—and fatter.

# Abdominal Etching

This is a relatively new technique. It could be called Lipo-lite, and it's for the abdomens of women who have decent stomachs but want better muscle definition. Abdominal etching is similar conceptually to using strategically applied self-tanning lotion or sprays that give the illusion of a six-pack. Abdominal etching sculpts your fat pads into a *trompe l'oeil* of chiseled abs. It's like a six-pack but non-alcoholic.

## How It's Done

Got an hour? That's all you'll need for a session of abdominal etching. Get yourself to a plastic surgeon's office. He'll give you a sedative and a local anesthetic—shots of lidocaine or another painkiller—in the gut. Then, he'll ask you to crunch your abs, what you've got of them, and draw a map of the natural musculature on your stomach. You will either lie down on a table or have the procedure standing upright. Next, the doc'll make tiny incisions in the navel for cannula insertion. Using the mini-tube, he'll suck out fat in grooves along the previously drawn guide of your ab muscles. It's like following a treasure map that leads him to your sculpted belly.

Post-op, give it a couple hours for the meds to wear off before you walk out of there. You'll have to sport a compression garment for a few weeks. Depending on your personal pain threshold, you might need drugs for a few days. No heavy lifting for a month.*

## What's This Gonna Cost Me?

If you get stomach lipo first, as many etching patients do, the price goes up. For a lipo/sculpt job, expect to pay no less than $5,000, and no more than $10,000. If you already have a decent belly and just want to create the appearance of definition, an ab etch only should run you approximately $2,500 to $5,000.

## Remind Me Again, Why Do I Want to Do This?

The rewards:

Ever looked at a picture of Jennifer Aniston's abs and felt a deep green envy rise in your throat? **Etching makes the envy go away.** You'll have (the appearance of) Jen's abs. Now only if you could have one night with John Mayer as she did. Maybe *then* you'll be happy.

## What's the Worst That Can Happen?

The risks:

**The usual grab-bag of side effects to the human body when you stick it with needles, knives, and metal tubes.** All of the risks are minimal but should be mentioned.

To prevent **infection,** you'll probably get antibiotics.

**Bleeding** is always a possibility. Your doctor will monitor it during surgery and give you warning signs to look for afterwards.

**Pain** is easily managed with pills.

*This is an excellent time to hire a maid.

**Scars** will be minimal, in the navel or along the stomach's natural creases.

**Swelling?** Wear the girdle.

**Bruising?** It'll fade in a few weeks.

**Lying to your friends to explain how you went from Dough Girl to American Gladiatrix overnight?** Don't lie! Tell the truth. It won't hurt you, and it might help them.

## LipoDissolve: Too Good to Be True?

During your lunch hour, you go to a spa, get some painless liquid injections, go back to work. A few days later, you've lost an inch around your waist. The so-called "lunchtime lipo" procedure, aka LipoDissolve or mesotherapy, sounds way too good to be true. Reports are mixed. The singer Roberta Flack claimed to have lost forty pounds after a year-long series of treatments. The news show "20/20" ran an expose on LipoDissolve that essentially called it a dangerous scam. Britney Spears allegedly tried it, and we all know what her stomach looks like these days—not exactly a ringing endorsement.

Regarding safety, the jury—or, I should say, FDA approval board—is out. There are no scientific studies that prove mesotherapy works or is safe. Meanwhile, thousands of willing Americans are putting themselves under the needle(s) anyway. Critics call it voluntary human experimentation.

The basics: mesotherapy has been around for fifty years. It's very popular in Europe (like Jerry Lewis, Mickey Rourke, and David Hasselhoff—reason enough to have doubts). The practice involves making scores of shallow injections into the mesodermal layer of skin. The chemical cocktail breaks down fat cell membranes and dissolves the fat, thereby causing weight loss and the disappearance of cellulite.

Each treatment requires dozens, even hundreds, of injections into the area. Large area, more injections. To guide him, the technician draws a grid pattern on your belly, say twenty rows of twenty dots about half an inch apart,* and injects the solution into each dot. To see optimal results (again, if the treatment works at all; we don't have proof it does), you need a series of four or more treatments, once every two or three weeks. Each treatment costs anywhere from $400 to $1,000. Expect to swell up for forty-eight hours after each visit. Proponents promise half an inch to an inch of reduction per treatment. Theoretically, after four treatments, your waist would go from a thirty-two to a twenty-eight.

Too bad there's no proof it actually works!

I'll tell you what frightens me most about mesotherapy: there's no standard solution. For all you know, the needles are full of gasoline. "Doctors" create their own formulas. You could go to five different spas and get five different cocktails of plant extracts, vitamins, enzymes, hormones, alpha lipid acids, and chemicals. One commonly used ingredient is phosphatidyl choline or PC, which can cause dangerous swelling and inflammation. The chemical is banned in Brazil, where plastic surgery is the national sport. Another is Lipostabil®, which causes swelling, lumps, and ulcerations. None of these drugs have been tested for short- and long-term effects. Some patients have reported bad scarring, necrosis (skin death), and severe allergic reactions. It sounds terrifying to me. This is a willy-nilly outpatient procedure without much—if any—monitoring of the patient's recovery or response to treatment. Meanwhile, all this fat that is allegedly broken down and dissolved? Where the hell does it *go*? Proponents say it's excreted from the body. In other, less delicate words, you poop it out. "The fat that is treated is allegedly broken down and dissolved by the action of the injected drugs. Proponents say it's excreted from the body. There is no completed study that addresses how the treated fat leaves the body," said Dr. Zevon.

If the fat dissolves (big if), it won't necessarily find its way into your

---

*Your stomach will look like Helen Keller's to-do list.

digestive system. It could just as well wind up in your lympathic system and eventually your cardiovascular system, where it might decide
to stay.

At least with liposuction, you know the fat is out of your body. With
LipoDissolve, you might be moving it from your butt and putting it in your
heart.

# Eleven

# Cutting Out the Middle

Joan had been working her way down in her makeover, and now she had literally reached the middle of her task. She had a bit of a belly, okay, a literal pouch had formed there that could carry a small family of kangaroos. And though she was an animal lover, she hated freeloaders and knew men were already scared away by women who were coming to the table with children, much less a small family of 'roos.

Stubbornly refusing the surgical route, she hatched a plan to banish the fat on her terms. She arrived at a theater in a tiny Cotswolds village in the English countryside that was home to a popular Japanese tourist attraction featuring actors in "Swinging '60s" costumes. Unfortunately for our heroine, her costume was a miniskirt with white go-go boots. As she was no Twiggy—more like Saggy—the Asian shutterbugs hid their cameras when they saw her. Joan knew something drastic had to be done. (Note to self: when the Japanese won't photograph you, something is terribly wrong.) Joan urgently phoned a plastic surgeon back home to schedule a tummy

*tuck or two. Unfortunately Star Jones had the week booked, but Joan was*
*able to get in the following week.*

In the hourglass that is my figure, most of the sand is stuck in the middle.

Actually, my boobs measure exactly the same as my waist, because my boobs *are* my waist.

I once complained to my husband about my belly fat, and he told me not to worry, because my breasts covered it.

A well-defined waist is often the most enviable body part in other women. Men like an itty-bitty waist. Across the globe, a tapered waist expanding into rounded hips is the key factor in a woman's sexual attractiveness. You could have the face of a dog, but if you've got the waist of a wasp, men will swarm toward you.

## Why Do Men Love Curves?

Some ideas:

1. **Curves are a sign of fertility.** From an evolutionary standpoint, the earliest cavemen made the empirical connection between a woman with good hips and childbearing. They also made a link between women with thick waists and their grandmothers.
2. **Curves are fun to drive.** Men love the metaphors that compare cars to women's bodies and sex to driving. The poet e.e. cummings, in his poem "she being Brand" describes a man driving a new, hard-to-handle car for the first time—a metaphor about deflowering a jittery virgin. And people think poetry is boring.
3. **Curves are dangerous.** Anything a man doesn't understand or possess is to be feared or coveted. We have

curves, they don't. Ergo, our figures are both intimidating and desirable.

4. **Curves are sexy.** That's really the point. Sexually speaking—and don't kid yourself, physical attractiveness is all about sex—most men adore a rounded, cushion-like bottom. However, without a trim waist to go with it, men won't think "cushion." They simply think "couch" and reach for the remote control.

# Waist to Hip

The percentage of the waist circumference to the hip circumference is known as your waist-to-hip ratio or WHR. Although you might've never heard of the WHR* before, it's a very important acronym. Even more important, according to scientists, than your BMI, or body mass index. Your BMI indicates how fat you are. But your WHR indicates how happy and healthy you are.

Along with being inundated with male attention, pear-shaped women (those with low WHRs) are smarter, more fertile, will live longer, will make more money, have bigger houses, wear nicer clothes, and drive better cars. Scientists have proven this! Most of it, anyway. I exaggerate for my own amusement. But I really did read about one study that found the children of small-waisted, ample-hipped mothers scored better on intelligence tests. It has to do with their having abundant quantities of polyunsaturated fat—the kind found in the butt and thighs—needed to feed the hungry fetal brain. And you thought your kid was a good student because she studies hard. Wrong. It's because you, and I mean this as compliment, have a big fat ass.

Conversely, apple-shaped women (those with high WHRs) have

*For years, I thought it was a radio station in Pittsburgh.

an increased risk for diabetes, heart disease, some cancers, obesity, infertility, and I might add spinsterhood, poverty, and general misery.

Fashion exists to emphasize the WHR. Even cavewomen cinched their wildebeest-hide dresses with decorative vines. In modern times, women have used bustles, hoop skirts, petticoats, corsets, and girdles to shrink the waist and boost the bottom. The corset alone is singularly responsible for propagation of the species during times of sexual repression.

Victorian England—a corseted era—was so repressed, it was considered uncouth to display the legs of a piano. Would Rhett Butler have given a damn about Scarlett O'Hara if it weren't for her eighteen-inch waist? Women used to pull corsets so tight that they were constantly swooning and fainting in warm rooms.

And it wasn't because they were delicate, fragile, sickly creatures!

The blood flow to their brains was cut off by the **lacing**.

Thousands of whales died to bone ladies' undergarments. Whales made women thin. Funny no one saw the irony of that. Until now.

If you're feeling adventurous and want to calculate your WHR, here's the step by step process:

1. Wrap a tape measure around the smallest part of your waist. Write down the number of inches.
2. Wrap the tape measure around the widest part of your hips. This is the only time you *want* your hips to be big, so you'll do yourself no favors by skimping.
3. Calculators out! Divide waist measurement by hip measurement. If, in your case, it's 26 divided by 36, that makes your waist-to-hip ratio 0.72. Same as Marilyn Monroe, Sophia Loren, and the Venus de Milo.

The ideal WHR for women, in terms of sexual attractiveness to men, is 0.7. For good health, it should be 0.8 or below. Higher than 0.85, expect to have a stern conversation with your doctor at your next checkup.

For men, the ideal WHR is 0.9. His hips and waist are almost the same measurement. Women, like men, are attracted to their opposite. A man with narrow hips and a big beer belly isn't defining sexy. But he's a bona fide hottie compared to a man with a small waist and a wide ass. Men with hips? Just thinking about it makes my last ovary shrivel.

Considering the desirability of a tiny waist, it should come as no surprise that abdominoplasty, aka the tummy tuck, was the fifth most popular plastic surgery in 2007. This procedure, usually in conjunction with strategic hate handle liposuction, flattened the bellies and cinched the waists of 148,000 patients last year. I'll bet they all tried their hardest to get a slender waist on their own. Dieting. Crunches. Sit-ups on that big rubber ball at the gym. The Ab-Lounger. You do what you can, but at a certain point, you hit a wall. And that wall is made of spare tire, hate handle, and belly fat that has no intention of going away quietly.

Is there anything more frustrating than belly fat?* Women who've been pregnant are especially vexed by the flabby skin on the midsection. They might be skinny everywhere else, but the belly looks stretched out like a deflated tire. Having a plump belly because of pregnancy is nothing to be ashamed of. It's a badge of horror—I mean honor!—to remind you what your body has been through. The sag of skin and extra padding, rest assured, is not your fault.

I had a tummy tuck about twenty years ago, as an adjunct to a hysterectomy. The ob/gyn surgeon removed my female bits, and then, in a move almost unheard of back then, I had a plastic surgeon come into the ER to finish the job.

I figured, if I'm going to be sliced open and have to endure that

*Aside from trying to find a cab driver in New York who speaks English.

non-elective operation, I might as well come out of it with a nice, tight tummy.

And it was the best thing I ever did. I was thrilled with how it looked. All the other women in the ward who had had hysterectomies were all going around crying and saying, "Boo-hoo, I'll never have any more children." And there I was smiling and saying, "I can't wait to get back in my bikini." What's more liberating than looking down and seeing a nice, flat stomach?

With the big-ticket operations, such as a tummy tuck, most women have some ambivalence and guilt to deal with beforehand. Why should you spend thousands of dollars and give up a month (or more) of your life to fix a problem surgically that can be corrected through sacrifice and suffering?

By "sacrifice and suffering," of course, I'm referring to "diet and exercise." Let me relieve you of your ambivalence now: *For mommies, the abdomen is largely immune to the effects of diet and exercise.*

When you're pregnant, your belly skin is stretched (this we know). Unless you're eighteen and have skin like a rubber band, it won't snap back to the way it was before. Multiple pregnancies sap the elasticity out of the stomach skin no matter how springy it once was. This is the price of pregnancy. We give our babies life; they give us sagging, loose, stretched-out skin.

Even Cindy Crawford, a mother of two, has fleshy puckering underneath her belly button, as seen in paparazzi bikini pictures. You can diet away fat, yes. But you can't diet away skin. The rest of your body could be as scrawny as a starved cat, but the stomach slack? Yours to keep.

What's more, your abdominal muscles—the six-pack—were stretched and separated during pregnancy. Picture them in two vertical rows of three little muscle rectangles, all nice and neat. (I think of them as ab-dominos.) When you expand during pregnancy, the two vertical rows are pulled apart. The technical term is "diastasis." Post-pregnancy, instead of the two, neat, tight, vertical rows of muscles, you have two curved parentheses, with a gap of nothing between them. That gap—which adds inches to your waist—can't be closed, no matter how many Pilates core classes you take. You could do a thousand crunches a day, and your waist still won't go back to its pre-pregnancy measurement.

Women who've never reproduced* but have a genetic pre-disposition to carrying their fat around the middle will also find relief via tummy tuck. I have a friend who runs marathons, is a vegetarian, never drinks beer, has never been pregnant, and yet, since she was ten years old, has had this little pouch. She's an ideal candidate for a tummy tuck.

Every doctor on our advisory panel wanted me to make it ab-solutely clear that a tummy tuck is not a weight-loss strategy: obese women, especially those with diabetes or heart problems, would put themselves at risk of a heart attack or a dangerous infection if they had a tummy tuck or any plastic surgery.

In fact, even if you're not obese, a lot of doctors would advise you to go on a diet and exercise plan *before* your surgery. Lose whatever weight you can first and then let them do the rest. Streamlining your body will streamline the operation.

## The Full Monty

To renovate the entire midsection, from rib cage to public bone, you'll need a full tummy tuck, most likely with a chaser of hate handle/belly liposuction.

The severity of an operation can be judged by recovery time. As a full tummy tuck is a major operation, it will take up to two months to fully recover. After a month, however, your belly will be so flat, you can bounce quarters, or a quarterback, off it. You could iron on it. Your waist will be wispy. Belt-worthy.

*like Minnie Mouse

## How's It Done?

Fair warning: Reading a description of the full tummy tuck isn't for the faint of stomach. If you're squeamish and wish to keep your lunch, skip ahead a few paragraphs.

The full tummy tuck is usually done under general anesthesia. Some mavericks will do it under a local, just numbing the area, as ob/gyn surgeons often do to perform caesarians. Personally, as during sex, I would rather be sound asleep.

Once you're under, the doctor will draw the dotted guidelines for the incisions. If you're having lipo too, you'll be marked where the cannula will be inserted. Because tumescent fluid needs to be inside the body for at least ten minutes, optimally forty minutes, before the fat can be suctioned away, doctors will usually infuse the area with the fluid first, then start making the tummy tuck incisions. After forty minutes or an hour of tummy tucking, they'll then return to the liposuction procedure to aspirate the fat.

Typically, for the full tummy tuck, the first cut is a curved line, from hip to hip, that runs below your stomach pouch and above the pubic bone. The second cut is a lollipop incision: a circle around the belly button and a vertical line straight down to the hip-to-hip incision.

Next, the doctor will use a cautery device and scissors or a scalpel to peel the large flaps of skin up and away from the muscle wall from pubic bone to rib cage.

Your abdominal wall is now exposed. Remember the two curved rows of muscles, the six-pack parentheses? Using a diagonal stitch, the doctor sews the rows of muscles back into their pre-pregnancy position.

It's like lacing sneakers and pulling them tight, narrowing the waist in the process. The sutures will dissolve on their own and won't need to be removed later on.

Next, it's time to drape the skin/fat layer tight over the tightened abdominal muscle wall. The excess skin will be trimmed. How much? "Let's say you have a patient who had gained weight in pregnancy and then returned to her weight prior to the pregnancy," said Dr. Zevon. "If there was fifteen centimeters of excess skin vertically, the optimal length of the incision would be forty-five centimeters for a three-to-one ratio. That allows there to be a smooth, flat scar without excess tissue, sometimes called 'dog ears,' at the end of the skin closure." The excised skin weighs a few pounds.

At this point (or before), the doctor will go back to the lipo part of the procedure and use a suction cannula to aspirate fat from the belly, hate handles, and, sometimes, the lower back.

If the operation were to end there, you'd have a flat belly and tighter waist, with one big problem: no belly button. The internal navel is where it used to be, but the hole opening had been part of the excised skin. Unless you want people to think you're a clone, the doctor then cuts a new hole in the skin, like opening a window for your navel to show through, and makes a circle of stitches to sew the navel to the hole of skin.

Next, the doctor will insert some drainage tubes into the abdomen and sew up the bottom incision. You'll have two scars—a long curved one running hip-to-hip, and a small round one encircling the new belly button. The drainage tubes will stay in place for a few days. You'll have to wear a girdle-type compression garment for a few weeks, too. The whole operation will last from three to five hours.

## The Mini Monty

A mini tummy tuck, unlike its big sister, is for women who have loose skin below the belly button only. No bulging upper-abdominal sag. A mini is for women, like my marathoner friend, who are skinny, except for the one infuriating roll between the navel and the pubic bone, or for women who have puckered, hanging skin from pregnancy that they have to tuck into their jeans like a shirt tail. The mini can take care of that, with less hassle and pain than a full. But, alas, it's still heavy-duty surgery. Any tummy tuck is significant—in time, money, and pain. Consider yourself warned.

## How's It Done?

For the mini tummy tuck, you'll be put under—or, for the brave, shot full of a local numbing agent. The surgeon will draw the dotted curved line just above the pubic bone and under your pouch. The mini-tuck incision is shorter—six to eight inches across—and the scar will be hidden entirely by your panties or a bikini bottom.

Once the incision has been made, the doctor will separate the skin/fat layer from the abdominal wall with a cautery device and a scalpel. He'll peel the skin upward to expose the vertical rows of muscle, aka the six-pack. But since he's working on the lower abdominal wall only, he'll be attending to only four of the muscles, which he'll suture closer together, using a criss-cross stitch, into neater vertical rows.

Again, it looks like lacing up a sneaker and pulling it tight.

Next, he'll pull the skin tightly back over the lower abdomen and cut off whatever hangs over the incision line. It's like hemming your stomach. He'll put some drainage tubes in the belly to prevent fluid accumulation, and then he'll close you up neatly. Since he worked on the lower region only, the belly button won't need to be repositioned. The operation will last three hours or so. You'll have to leave the drains in for a few days, as well as wear a girdle-esque garment to prevent swelling.*

---

*The glamour never ends.

## What's This Gonna Cost Me?

For a full tummy tuck, you're looking at as little as $6,000 and as much as $15,000. It's a huge range. If you're getting liposuction of the belly and/or hate handles along with the tuck, expect a quote at the high end of the range. For a mini, the range is smaller: $5,000 to $8,000. Remember, you're paying for the surgeon, the facility, the anesthesiologist, the nurses and assistants, the meds (before, during, and after surgery), the follow-up care.* For any major cosmetic surgery, expect to pay $5,000 just to walk in the door.

## Remind Me Again, Why Do I Want to Do This?

The rewards:

**A week recuperating.** If you've got enough magazines, dirty novels, and romantic comedies, a week's time-out shouldn't be too taxing. For the first two days, you won't be able to stand up. Let your staff of servants (aka, your friends and family) cater to your every whim. It's only temporary.

**Two months' gym reprieve.** No strenuous exercise for two months? No problem! Next time you hit the gym, all the regulars will be amazed by your new body. Tell them that, instead of working out, you sat on your ass for eight weeks, and look what happened.

**No more trapeze tops.** Sick to death of bubble dresses and swing jackets? After your tummy tuck, say good-bye to Lane Bryant separates. You'll be shopping for body-clinging, tight, form-fitting dresses, blouses, and blazers that would look good on Ashlee Simpson. After years of dressing to camouflage your mid-section, you can now set it free. Go ahead, show an inch of skin above your pants.

**Confidence.** Nothing makes you feel quite as secure as walking down the street with the utter confidence that your stomach is not

---

*Not to mention alimony payments for your doctor's second and third ex-wives.

jiggling. Or to pose for a photo without hiding your gut behind a briefcase or a purse or a midget friend. After a tummy tuck, you can put yourself front and center.

## What's the Worst That Can Happen?

The risks:

**Death.** With any procedure that requires general anesthesia, there's a 1 in 100,000 chance of going to sleep and never waking up. A tummy tuck is major surgery and should be considered with the proper gravity.

**Infection.** Another omnipresent risk when you're being cut into, your insides exposed to the air, tools, gloved hands. I've heard several doctors say the risk of infection is why going to a private office surgical facility is actually safer than going to a hospital where there are sick people and germs. Make sure the facility is AAAASF-accredited (American Association for Accreditation of Ambulatory Surgery Facilities). Pre- and post-op, just to be sure, you'll probably get antibiotics anyway.

**Bleeding/embolism.** During surgery, the doctor will cauterize the cut vessels to prevent internal bleeding. But he might miss a few. Most bleeders stop on their own. If not, the doctor might have to go back in to take care of it. Check for excessive bruising and swelling—beyond what you can normally expect. Also, a bubble of air can sneak its way into a vessel. If the bubble reaches your brain or lungs, that would be bad. Both risks are rare.

**Swelling/bruising.** The drainage tubes and compression garment keep swelling and discoloration under some control. But you should still expect a lot of both. You've been cut wide open, after all. Your blood and lymph systems will rush to your defense, whether you want their help or not. Swelling is part of healing. The drains come out after a few days. Fluids start to recede after two weeks. By the end of three months, it's 90 percent gone. As far as the bruising, your skin will be normal in color after six weeks, if not sooner.

**Pain.** Doctors liken the pain of a tummy tuck to that of a caesarian. You may experience muscle cramps. Achingly tight skin. Not being able to stand upright for a week. The chafing from drainage tubes. Ice packs and the compression garments help a little. Pain meds help a lot. This is not the time to be prudent or "brave." Take the pills! Be prudent and brave next week. And be sure to blame it on your kids. Again.

**Numbness.** Prepare for spotty numbness on the surface of your skin around the incision area. Usually, sensation returns after a month. Sometimes, it's gone for good.

**Scarring.** There will be permanent scars. No sugar-coating the reality of tummy tucking. For the full treatment, the scar will run hip to hip. Mine was along the bikini line, and eventually turned white and all but disappeared. Also, you'll have a ring-shaped scar around your new belly button. If you have a good surgeon and good skin, it's virtually invisible after it's healed. Even in the best of all possible worlds, though, you don't always get a perfect outcome.

Patricia "Everyone Loves Plastic Surgery" Heaton, mother of four, admitted to having had a tummy tuck. She didn't do so well with her scars, especially around her herniated navel, which appeared to have folded over itself. She still said she'd recommend a tummy tuck to anyone.

"There is no way to guarantee how the scar will look in any particular individual," said Dr. Scott Zevon. "You can do the same procedure on different people and get a different-quality scar. There is an element of scar maturation that's out of the surgeon's control. If someone has multiple scars that have healed poorly without due cause, the surgeon would raise the possibility that they will scar poorly again."

**Disappointment.** You thought you'd be a goddess, but turned out to be You, Only Better. Maybe you thought your stretch marks would disappear. FYI: stretch marks on the excised skin are gone from your life forever. Others, on your sides, for instance, won't be fixed via tummy tuck. After all that pain and money, you do not have the belly of your dreams. This is why doctors chant the phrase "realistic expectations." With all treatments and surgeries, you're paying for visible *improvement*. A tummy tuck will definitely improve the appearance of your stomach. It won't miraculously transform you into Beyoncé.

No matter how much money you spend, you are still you. Which is exactly how it should be.

## Combining Tummy Tuck with Other Surgeries

Maybe you've heard about the Mommy Makeover: a combination of procedures for women whose body parts suffered during pregnancies. Perhaps the breasts got big during nursing and then deflated. Or the once narrow waist stretched out during pregnancy, and extra skin around the middle hangs off your formerly flat stomach. Your friendly neighborhood plastic surgeon will be happy to put that bounce back in your boobs and the tight back in your tummy all in one shot, a double-whammy job. It's a full day on the table—a minimum of six hours—and it's a major hit on your bank account, cost starting at $15,000. The recovery isn't easy. You'll be chin to crotch in bandages. Maybe it should be called the Mummy Makeover. You won't be able to lift anything heavier than a pint of ice cream for a month post-op: make sure that your husband/lover/ the bastard who got you pregnant is available to get the kids in and out of car seats and the bathtub. I would urge anyone to wait for a full year after you've finished breast-feeding your last kid to do this.

This double-whammy procedure is one example of the new trend of having two or more major plastic surgeries in one shot. The theory is that you save money by paying for anesthesia only once. Indeed, most doctors will give multiple-procedure discounts. Also, you get it all over with quickly. Although the recovery might be twice as painful by doing a lot of surgery at once, it'll take half as long as staging two procedures over time.

"At some point it is likely that there is a greater risk with combined procedures than of the abdominoplasty alone but not necessarily greater than the risks of the two procedures performed at different times," said Dr. Zevon. "There comes a point where you want to stage operations done on an ambulatory basis. I'd say six hours is the maximum." Surely, surgery that long takes a physical toll on the surgeon, as well? "Performing surgery can be relaxing," Dr. Zevon says.

Personally, I like the small-tweaks approach. God knows, I've had a lot done over the years, but I chose to do it a little at a time. Doing an extreme makeover involves six hours of anesthesia—*at least*—and cutting into multiple body parts all in one day. That scares me, and it can be a major shock to the body.*

The best of all possible worlds? I saw an ad on Craig's List recently, posted by a plastic surgeon in the Hamptons, offering the June to September rental of his beachfront mansion, as well as all the plastic surgery the renter desires, for the price of $500,000. What could be better? Staggering procedures every couple of weeks, recuperating in a beautiful setting, under the twenty-four-hour care of your surgeon? A summer of rebirth on the beach! It sounds like a little bit of heaven, for whoever can afford it.

---

*Like the time I heard that Tom Cruise has sex with women.

# The Knife-Free Tummy Tuck

The days of death-defying undergarments—corsets that cut off circulation to the brain and girdles that caused internal injury—are over. Or are they? We've entered a new era, people. The Era of Shapewear.

Body shapers, garments that pack you in tighter than sausage casing, aren't brand spanking new in the world of fine washables, but they've certainly gone mainstream again. Celebs like Gwyneth Paltrow, Jessica Alba, Oprah Winfrey all swear by these products. Some of the options are footless hose for jeans, regular hose, magic panties, smoothing bras, slimming camisoles, leotard-like body suits, body shapers that go up to the bra and down to the thighs, bike shorts–style tummy/hip huggers.

My verdict on shapewear? Meh. They're good, but not great. Okay, who doesn't want to put on a newfangled girdle and look like you've instantly lost five to ten pounds? Undeniably, you do look better inside the sausage casing. Lumps look less, but you've still got them!

Also, let's not forget the difficulty just to get the body shaper *on*. It's high. Last time I crammed myself into one—like getting toothpaste inside a tube—I almost broke a hip. I started sweating and had to redo my makeup. I pulled it halfway up and got stuck.

I had to call the fire department to bring over the jaws of life. The firemen arrived, got one look at me and, instead of breaking the door down, they started to barricade me in.

Seriously, the body shapers are great for slacks, sheath dresses, an evening gown—if you're standing up. I wear them on the red carpet. But when I go inside and take my seat, the high-waisted kind of garment often rolls down to my waist. It's supposed to stay up, right under the bra. You can sew it to your bra, effectively locking yourself into it. The Spanx body shaper has a strap that hooks onto the bra to keep it up, but it isn't enough. Also, the ass/hip shapers compress your parts into a bizarre circular uni-butt.

If you do catch a man's attention and bring him home, keep in mind that your body shaper looks good *under* clothes, but it is *not* sexy alone. I have a friend who let a guy undress her down to her body shaper. She excused herself to the bathroom to struggle out of it in private indignity. When she emerged three hours later, he was gone.

When she confronted him the next day, he said the body shaper reminded him of his grandmother who was buried wearing one.

## ( Twelve )

# Eyes Wide Open

*All of this beauty maintenance begins to take a toll on a person if they are not careful, and Joan was no exception. She was beginning to look perpetually tired because of the heavy bags underneath her eyes. They were so big that her mother gave her luggage tag earrings for her birthday. Joan knew from experience that Preparation H helped shrink puffiness. She also realized that in New York and LA finding Preparation H would be difficult since there were so many assholes in need of shrinkage.*

*Luckily, she had a Plan B. Two flights and three camel rides later, Joan arrived in the Middle East wearing a black, shapeless burka with only a tiny slit for her eyes to peer out. It perfectly concealed the problem, and while she was covered head to toe in a garment no one would ever call a "dude magnet" (but then again who wants to attract the likes of these dudes—if that's what she wanted, she would have just hailed a cab and flirted with the driver the entire way), it was a small price to pay to keep her eye bags out of the public's view. It wasn't until she hopped off the camel's back that she remembered how much she hated getting sand in her shoes at the beach, the oppression of women, and food that looked like it came out of the hind end of a dromedary. These were the deal-breakers that sent her home to the air-conditioned suites of a plastic surgeon who performed eye jobs and served her tea. When Joan accidentally spilled some of the tea on his plush carpet, he didn't even suggest her hands be cut off, and at that moment she knew she made the right decision to come back to the United States and get this procedure.*

Cross into your fifties, and you become the invisible woman (unless you live in Florida; there, you're a spring chicken). It's like you're incognito, without wanting to be. Being old is like wearing Harry Potter's Cloak of Invisibility, all the time. A good way to tear it off is an eye lift. As one of my doctors (can't remember which, there've been so many) used to say, "When you hit fifty, you need a liftie."*

You've heard that the eyes are the window to the soul? Wrong. For a peek at someone's soul, get a load of his tax return, under the category of charitable donations. Or watch how he treats animals, the elderly, and children. Or cut him off in traffic.

The eyes are not the windows to but the mirrors of the soul. When you glance in the mirror and see saggy, tired, puffy eyes, your soul plummets to the floor. It's hard to feel young and vital when you know you look ancient and tired (and I mean that in the nicest possible way). The way your eyes appear—heavy, droopy, and exhausted—turns into the way you feel and behave.

It's a crime, what aging does to the eyes. Once upon a time, when introduced to, for example, your boss's daughter who, poor child, was born with all the beauty and charm of a pig, you'd say, "What lovely eyes you have!" Come age fifty, the lovely-eyed among us can't rightfully expect to hear even the lowest form of left-handed compliment. It's like robbing a beggar of her last dollar.

---

*Thank God his surgical skills were better than his jokes.

Sunglasses help. Anna Wintour, editor-in-chief of *Vogue*, clued into this decades ago, as did Jackie O. Both ladies decided that camouflage was the way to go, put on a pair of big, black sunglasses and had them surgically attached to their faces. A temporary and slightly uncomfortable fix. Eventually, both Anna and Jackie, allegedly, got a blepharoplasty, otherwise known (affectionately) as the eye lift.

Over 241,000 other women did so in 2007, making it the fourth most popular surgical procedure of the year.

## Look Me in the Eye

Having awake-looking eyes isn't only crucial for feeling alive in our own souls. We communicate with our eyes. They tell the world more about what we're thinking and feeling than even our lips.

Try to be coquettish with your cheekbones. Try to seduce a man using your nostrils. Not even Kathleen Turner, in her heyday, could do it.

Most of us need the help of our sexy bedroom eyes, a flutter of lashes, a glint, a gleam. But when your lids are so heavy that just keeping them open is a chore, you can't possibly muster a flutter. Your glint is obscured by puffiness. The gleam? Dulled by loose skin.

The sad reality? Your bedroom eyes have turned into bathroom eyes. Down the toilet.

And what about boardroom eyes? You need the steady eye contact and stare-down seriousness that communicate self-assuredness and confidence. Who can pull that off when your eyes look like Abe Vigoda's? How can you get your message to the world when your lids are hiding your intentions?

Along with a sexy glimpse and a steely glare, the eyes communicate a huge range of meaning, all of which might be lost for the lid-challenged. Here are some "tells" of the eye, according to people who make a living studying facial movements (FYI: the directionals are for righties; lefties can just put them in reverse):

1. **When you look up and to the right,** it means you're flashing back to a place memory, like the last half-off sale at Neiman Marcus.
2. **When you look up and to the left,** you're drawing a picture in your head, like wondering what sex would be like if your husband stayed awake during it.
3. **When you look to the right,** you're recalling a conversation that actually happened, like when you described to your shrink your recurring sexual fantasy about Johnny Depp and an edible jockstrap.
4. **When you look to the left,** you're thinking of a conversation you wished you'd had, like how you shouldn't have replied when the waiter asked, "Would you ladies care for dessert?"
5. **When you look down and to the right,** you're talking to yourself, say, about how much you deserve an eye lift.
6. **When you look down and to the left,** you're tasting something from the past.
7. **When you look straight ahead,** and then over to the right, while sticking your middle finger out the window, you're driving.
8. **When you look up, then down, then to the right, then to the left,** you're flirting, which would work much better if you were a) ten years younger, or b) *looked* ten years younger after an eye lift.

The eyes have it. And "it," as far as I can see, is the ability to seduce, beguile, and connect with other people. More than any other feature on your face, the eyes do the heavy lifting of communication. Sadly, they also do the heavy lifting of bags and sags. You want the person sitting across from you to focus on the intensity and passion in your gaze. Not whether you've slept in the past two months.

# Upper Eyelid

Redundant skin. That's what surgeons call the hood of skin that takes over the upper eye lids as you get older. What causes the sag? Your tiny eye muscles weaken, as does the natural collagen and elastic fibers in your skin. Without tight skin and strong muscles to hold it in place, the adipose tissue that cushions the eye sockets slides down and accumulates. That's right. You *gain* weight—in your eyelid.

The visual effect? Like a hypnotist told you, "You are getting sleepy, very sleepy . . ." and then he left the party without snapping his fingers to wake you up.

It's disheartening, to say the least, when you feel alive and happy but look exhausted and depressed. Your eyelids themselves *are* tired. They have to hold up all that extra fat and skin with feeble muscles. Unfortunately, your eyelids can't go to the gym and pump iron to get stronger. And they can't go on a low-carb diet to lose weight.

The surgical approach to lifting the upper eyelid is pretty straightforward. You just have to get over two things, psychologically speaking: 1) a doctor will be sticking a knife within millimeters of your eyeball, and 2) a doctor will be sticking a knife within millimeters of your *other* eyeball.

Some people can get very squeamish about their eyes. I knew a woman who hated wearing glasses with a passion, but she was also deathly afraid of anything touching her eyes, including contact lenses. Whenever she tried to put them in, she broke out in a sweat and had a panic attack. Eventually, she got laser vision correction. The only way she could handle that procedure was to take enough Valium to sedate an elephant.

Be prepared that eye surgery is delicate. It's tender. And it's done, usually, with a local anesthetic. You will be awake—though numbed and sedated—while the doctor comes at your eyes with the blade, à la Freddy Krueger.

## How It's Done

First step, the doctor will draw an oval along the fold of the upper eyelid as an incision guide. He'll then give you local or, possibly, general anesthesia. When you're numb or asleep (my personal favorite), he'll use tiny surgical scissors and a scalpel to excise the previously marked strip of skin of the lid.

Once the skin is removed, the doctor will cut a smaller oval out of the underlying muscle layer to expose the orbital septum. The orbital septum is a thin membrane that holds the eye and its connective tissue in place, like a Ziploc plastic baggie filled with Jell-O. Your doctor will next make small slits into the baggie to access the two fat deposit areas of the upper lid.

The doctor presses on the eyelid to force the fat out of the membrane. Then, he'll clamp the fat clump, cut off some of it, and let the rest recede into the orbital septum. He won't take it all. You need a little fat in there to cushion the eyeball. Next, your doctor will stitch your skin back together nice and tight so that the sutures are right in the crease of the lid. He'll put some ointment and a teeny bandage on top, and you're done. Take a deep breath. Then he'll move over to the other eye.

The upper eyelid lift, both of them, will take an hour, tops. You'll walk out with no need for blinders or heavy *Pirates of the Caribbean* patches.

## Lower Eyelid

This procedure can be done under local or general anesthesia. Two ways to get rid of the twelve-piece set of bags you're carrying around under your eye. First, the transcutaneous approach, meaning going in from the outside. The first step: Your eye will be temporarily stitched closed. Next, the doctor will make an incision along the length of the lower lid, right under the lashline. Later, you can easily hide faint scars with makeup.

Next, he'll cut a hole in the muscle layer, and then using surgical tweezers, he'll pull back the skin and muscle to access the orbital septum, aka the membrane that holds the eye package in place.

Then, he'll cut a line in the orbital septum to get at the three fat deposits of the lower lid. The doctor will extract the fat, snip off some of it, cauterize where he cut to make sure it doesn't bleed, and then let what's left recede into the orbital septum. He'll then move to excess skin removal. To judge how much skin has to come off, the doctor may ask you to look up. If you chose general anesthesia, he'll have asked you to do this beforehand and marked the incision lines with a pen. As with upper-eyelid surgery, the doctor will cut away a sliver of extra skin and stitch you up tighter. And you're done, except for the other eye.

Doing both of them will take an hour or two. The extra risk with this approach is the lower eyelid healing too low and showing the iris all the way around.

The other lower-lid lift method is called transconjunctival, meaning getting in through the inside of the lid. The lower eyelid will be held open with a retractor. The conjunctiva, the pink part on the inside of the eyelid, is thereby made accessible. You might have a contact-like shield put on your eye to protect it before the doctor makes a horizontal cut along the conjunctiva to get at the three fat deposits in the lower lid.

He'll clamp and cut off a chunk of the fat, cauterize what's left to prevent bleeding, and then let the remainder sink back from whence it came. He'll do it for all three deposits.

Then, he'll remove the protective shield on the eye and ease up on the retractor. You won't get any stitches in the conjunctiva. No sewing means a faster procedure time and slightly lower cost.

## What's This Gonna Cost Me?

Depends, as usual, on where you have it done, your surgeon's experience, and exactly how much skin/muscle/fat needs to be removed. On average, according to the American Society of Plastic Surgeons, eye lifts cost $2,800 per lid pair. As usual, depending on where you live, you can expect to pay double that amount. If you're having the upper and lower lids done, expect to pay *no less* than $5,600.

## What's the Worst That Can Happen?

The risks:

You'll have **bruising** and **swelling** after surgery and look like you've gone five rounds with Evander Holyfield. (If anyone asks about it, just say, "You should've seen the other guy.") After a month, 80 percent of it will be gone. After three months, you'll have seen the last of it. And it's easy to cover with makeup.

**Scarring.** It'll be minimal and well placed, but be aware that you will have faint lines forever. They'll fade and are easily disguised with liner and shadow.

**Bleeding.** There's a chance that a cut vessel may leak, causing the dread hematoma, or bleeder. If you have unusual or disturbing swelling, call your doctor. He might have to suction out the blood with a syringe or go back in and cauterize the vessel.

**Dry eyes.** If too much skin is removed, and what's left of the lid is stretched paper thin, you might have a chronic dry eye problem. If drops don't help, the surgical fix is a skin graft on the eyelid.

**Blurry vision.** Immediately after surgery, you might have blurry vision. Do not freak out! It's only due to having had your eyes fiddled with for an hour or two. If your vision doesn't clear after a day or two, call your doctor.

## Remind Me Again, Why Do I Want to Do This?

The rewards:

**You'll look younger, more refreshed.**

Suddenly, other **people will see the real you.** The alive, happy, beautiful you that used to be hiding behind puffy, sleepy, heavy lids.

**People will stop handing you cups of coffee,** saying, "This will keep you awake."

**Increased visibility.** When you were twenty, thirty, forty, people gave you the proper attention when you walked into a store or restaurant.

**You can wear mascara again,** without it smudging on your puffy upper lid.

**When you take off your sunglasses,** no one asks if you stuck your face inside a beehive.

### Knife-Free Eye Lifts

Although surgery will net you the best, longest-lasting results, you don't have to go under the blade to perk up your lids. Any number of creams are for sale that make the old hope-in-a-jar promises. Maybe you've already tried—and been disappointed by—all the potions and lotions, but aren't quite ready yet for a surgical intervention. Fine. Great. You've got a few no-cut methods to choose from. They are:

**Fillers.** Great for the lower lid bags. Your doctor or dermatologist will inject Restylane or Juvéderm—hyaluronic acid fillers—to plump up the line under the bag. The basic idea is, if you fill the valley, the mountain disappears. The whole procedure will take less than an hour, cost less than $1,000, and last six to eight months.

**Radiothermoplasty.** A newish treatment option for skin resurfacing, radiothermoplasty—also known as ThermaLift®, Thermage®, or

ThermaCool®—uses high-frequency radio waves to heat up the collagen deep inside the dermis layer of your skin, while at the same time cooling the surface skin, or epidermis. The heated dermis contracts and tightens, and spurs the growth of new collagen for extra snap. The cooled epidermis doesn't burn, change pigment, or peel (although you will probably have temporary redness). The results? You'll have to wait up to six months to see them, unfortunately, because new collagen, alas, doesn't grow overnight. Once the swelling goes down in a week, though, you'll see your fine lines have disappeared, and your deeper crow's feet will improve daily. You'll enjoy the results for up to two years. Cost is high, about $1,000 to $5,000 per treatment. Not too much less than surgery.

**Laser resurfacing.** A nice idea for just the eye area, but people do get their whole face, neck, belly, chin, resurfaced with a laser, either a carbon-dioxide, Erbium: YAG, or a combo of the two. Your doctor will decide which laser in his holster would work best on your eye area. First, he'll numb the area and then wave the laser wand over the wrinkled and saggy skin. You might need just a few quick pulses or several longer hits, depending on the condition of the skin. The laser will destroy the top layers of skin. That will peel away and expose the undamaged, unwrinkled layers below. It's like taking off your middle-aged mask, to reveal the youthful beauty underneath. Along with a new surface, the deep skin layers, thanks to the laser's heat, will collagen up, adding firmness over time. You'll definitely have pain and swelling. The treatment area will be red and crusty for the better part of two weeks. It might stay a little red for *months*. But once the dead skin peels away, and your color returns to its normal hue, you'll be fresh and glowing—for up to two years. Warning! This ain't cheap. For only one treatment, it's around $2,500. You might need a few treatments.

I don't like the long recovery time. Also, only fair-skinned people can do it. If you're medium or dark, the laser could cause hyperpigmentation, or make your skin darker in spots.

# Forehead Lifts

If you have saggy upper lids as well as a thick cavewoman forehead, you might do even better than blepharoplasty by getting a brow lift, whereby your forehead is pulled back and sutured behind the hairline. It lifts your lids and forehead, and gets rid of the pesky lines between your eyebrows, the vertical crinkles around the brows, and the horizontal forehead gouges. In me, those crinkles were so deep that rock climbers used to get lost in them. I could've planted potatoes in them.

Botox Cosmetic injection can achieve a similar result, but a brow lift won't need to be refreshed every four months. This is a permanent solution to upper-face wrinkles, including frown lines and concentration lines, which I call punch lines (minus the humor). When they appear, I know it's time for a surgical punch-up.

As with the eyelids, the forehead droops as you age due to weakening muscles and stretched-out collagen in the deep skin layers. A brow lift won't strengthen the muscles or regrow collagen, though. Rather, it's like pulling the sheets tight on a bed and smoothing out a lumpy mattress.

Kathy Griffin had this done and said it made her look "months younger."

Seriously, it opened up her face and made her look younger and brighter.

Forty-three thousand people had forehead lifts in 2007, so Kathy wasn't alone. She probably had the traditional procedure, called a **coronal brow lift.**

## How It's Done

It's called a coronal lift because the incision is made across the crown of the scalp, or where WASPs wear their velvet headbands.

The pre-surgery prep will include making a nice wide part, from ear to ear, in your hair about an inch or two back from the hair line. The hair in front will be tied up in a dozen or so tiny ponytails to keep it out of the way.

Most doctors recommend general anesthesia. When you're asleep, the doctor will make an incision along the headband line, all the way across. Ear to ear. Next, he'll use a forceps and scissors to separate (or elevate) the skin and muscle away from the skull. For extreme lifts, the entire front scalp will be elevated, from the top of your head, to the temples on both sides, and as low as the eyebrow ridge. The flap of scalp is pulled down over your eyes and nose like a veil.

What your doctor sees: the underside of your forehead, including the three main muscle groups. The frontalis muscles are across the upper forehead. The procerus muscles are between the eyes. The brow's got corrugator muscles.

The next part of the brow lift operation is to disrupt the action of these muscles. The doctor will cut away small strips of the frontalis, procerus, and corrugator muscles, essentially disabling them. The removal of only tiny bits of the muscles prevents you from making certain facial movements—the ones that cause wrinkles—but not all movement. You'll lose the wrinkles but not your expressiveness. Win-win.

Onward to sewing your face back on. The doctor next pulls the scalp flap back up over the forehead. He'll pull the skin tight, gauging the appropriate level of tension. You'll have about a centimeter of excess skin to trim. When that's done, the doctor will close the incision, from ear to ear, giving you a new hairline. The stitches will be bandaged. You may or may not have a drainage tube in your temple. In a week, you can go back to work.

Just be careful you don't end up with that perpetually "surprised look" like House Speaker Nancy Pelosi—who seems to be in a constant state of astonishment.

But if you get a good brow lift, they'll wonder how you lost ten years and a lifetime of anxiety during your one-week vacation.

Since the hairline is yanked back, this isn't a good idea for women with high hairlines. Queen Elizabeth I, for example, couldn't have done this. Her hairline was already coronal high. Also, if you happen to be thinning on top, brow lifts leave an obvious scar.

The modified version of the coronal brow lift is the **endoscopic brow lift,** a relatively new procedure that uses super-cool gizmos and high-tech gadgets along with the old-school scalpels and sutures.

First off, you'll have general anesthesia. The hair along the hairline will be sectioned into tiny ponytails to keep it out of the way. The area along your hairline and scalp will be cleaned. Instead of the long incision, for this procedure the doctor will make three to five small holes in the scalp an inch behind the hairline. Through each hole, the doctor will slide blunt forceps back and forth, up and down, to detach the skin from the bone. The skin is loosened on the inside with the forceps.

Once the skin/muscle tissue is elevated from the bone, the doctor next inserts an endoscope through one of the holes. An endoscope is a surgical tool that allows doctors to see what's going on inside the body. It's a tube with a light and lens on the end (hence, end-o-scope) that's hooked up to a TV monitor. Once inserted through the incision holes, the doctor can see on TV what he's doing underneath the forehead skin.* He'll leave the endoscope in one of the holes to see and insert special forceps into another to cut away little bits of muscle—under the furrows, between the eyebrows, and just over the eyebrows. Shaving strips off the muscles disables them, preventing the micro-movements that cause wrinkles. So you lose the wrinkles but not most of your expressions.

Muscles successfully handicapped, the doctor next removes the forceps and endoscope, and proceeds to raise your forehead skin higher to get rid of that droopy brow better suited to Cro-Magnons and former East German beauty queens. Most likely, the doctor will

---

*As long as he hasn't already switched over to "Project Runway."

use stiches to hoist your forehead a few notches tighter. He might put in little implants that'll attach to the skull and hold the skin in a higher new position. In either instance, the sewing is limited to the incisions he'd already made. No major cutting needed.

After the sewing comes the bandaging. Then, you're sent on your way (with an escort, of course). The job, start to finish, will take one to three hours. There's a lot less cutting with an endoscopic lift, which speeds recovery time and healing. The effect will last until gravity takes hold of your forehead again—probably many years.

## What's This Gonna Cost Me?

The national average is around $3,000, but you can pay a whole lot more, up to $7,000. A endoscopic brow lift will be at the lower end of the range, and the coronal brow lift will be at the higher end.

## Remind Me Again, Why Do I Want to Do This?

The rewards:

With a nicely pulled brow, **you no longer look like a serial killer . . .**

Or **a cavewoman . . .**

Or **a brooding poet . . .**

Or **your perpetually pissed-off mother-in-law.**

You do look wide awake, fresh and unlined, young and alert, and ready for your next adventure.

## What's the Worst That Can Happen?

The risks:

**Bleeding/Infection.** By now, you know that there's a risk of bleeding and infection in any surgery. If you do bleed—you can tell by the excessive skin discoloration and weird, localized swelling—the pool can be drained with a needle or fixed with a second operation. Infection? Well, this is the twenty-first century, and doctors know how to treat such things. Usually, you'll get antibiotics before and after surgery to insure that you don't get one.

**Bruising/Swelling.** By now, you also know that when a doctor cuts muscle, you will bruise. You will swell. Depending on how drastic the lift, you'll be bruised/swollen for at least a week, maybe as many as four.

**Pain.** The swelling adds to the painful feeling of too-tight skin. This discomfort won't last long, a week or so, and you'll be given pain pills. You can safely go back to work after seven days and exercise/lift heavy objects (like a vibrator) within a month.

**Numbness.** You've got a lot of nerves in the face, and some of them might be bruised, stretched, or otherwise damaged during the procedure. Usually, any numbness will go away within a month of surgery.

**Scarring.** Unless you go bald or your hairline recedes, all your scars will be safely hidden in your hairline. They'll fade over time, too, but they are yours to keep, forever and ever.

**Disappointment.** A bad brow lift makes you look like you've been trapped in a wind tunnel. Or locked into a G-force simulator. You might decide that your new hairline is way too high or that your eyebrows are floating weirdly in the middle of your forehead. Avoid disappointment by communicating your desires exactly to your doctor. Say, "I want my eyebrows to end up here." Draw a picture or edit a photograph. And don't decide you absolutely hate the result until the swelling is completely gone—at least a few months.

## Prick Up Your Ear

Attention, Alfred E. Neuman and George W. Bush: Boing-boing ears can be fixed via a procedure called **otoplasty.** The ear job is usually done on children as young as four years old. The younger the better, to save them from years of being called Dumbo or Jughead at school.

In a procedure that takes up to three hours, the doctor cuts a slit in back of the ear, sections excess cartilage, and then sews it back together and into a new position closer to the head, sometimes sewing the back of the ear to the side of the head to train them. You'll have to wear a bandage, like a goofy headband, for a week or until the sutures dissolve.

And speaking of ears, another popular procedure can fix **huge holes or torn earlobes.** Heavy earrings are usually to blame for stretching out the holes. God forbid they get caught in your sweater as your date (hopefully) yanks it over your head, and—yowch!—blood, cartilage, skin turned to hamburger meat. Making a stretched-out earring hole smaller or reconnecting a split or torn earlobe is a minor surgery. It's done in the doctor's office, with local anesthesia. Takes less than an hour and costs only $400 to $1,000. Here's the scoop on earlobes: the doctor opens the skin on the inside of the torn flaps of the earlobe, then sews the flaps together. In two weeks, they'll have fused back into one piece. The stitches will dissolve on their own. You can get your ear pierced again, too, in a few months.

And next time, take your earrings off *before* the sweater.

# Celeb Eye Job and Brow Lift Ticker

Can't accurately say who's had a *good* upper face lift, be it eye or brow, since the best ones are subtle and just make you look fresh and awake. The bad eye jobs, however, are glaringly painful to behold.

## In the "Human or Vulcan?"* category:

**Kenny Rogers:** He might know when to hold 'em, know when to fold 'em, but he sure didn't know when to walk away from the operating table.

**Joan Van Ark.** Her eyebrows are halfway to the moon.

**Cher.** Well, she always looked out of this world. Now she looks perpetually surprised. Ask her how she is—she looks stunned. Ask her what she had for breakfast—she looks stunned. Ask her what time it is—she looks . . . well, you get the idea.

## In the "Yanked Back the Wig" category:

**Liza Minnelli.** Love her. She's a huge talent. And now she's got the huge forehead to go with it.

**Jessica Lange.** Beautiful woman. In her prime, she was almost alien gorgeous. Still looks good, except her forehead is two inches higher than it used to be.

## In the "Stapled Open" category:

**Bruce Jenner.** At nearly sixty, he's got the eyes of a twenty-year-old. The effect? Olympic weirdness.

**Sylvester Stallone.** Eyes stapled open, to match his mouth.

*Feel free to Google Leonard Nimoy and/or Mr. Spock.

( **Thirteen** )

# Arm and a Leg

After her tummy tuck, Joan was ready to shop for a bathing suit (every woman's darkest hour). She was feeling confident that her makeover was beginning to take form and that this experience would be different than the ones she had had in the past.

Unfortunately, the minute Joan got into a cute little rhinestone-accented tankini, she became aware of the multicolored patterns on her calves. In the past, Joan had thought her veined legs added character, and she had actually spent one summer putting the intricate web to good use by tutoring history students. Joan found that when she put her legs side by side, they actually resembled the map that Lewis and Clark used to mount their expedition across the United States.

Unfortunately, standing in the dressing room looking at herself in the bathing suit, Joan realized that the vein that represented the Missouri River had recently forked, and she knew this summer it would give students the mistaken impression that Sacagawea had led Lewis and Clark not to

*Oregon but rather to Brooklyn. Fearful that the entire class would flunk their make-up exams because of her, Joan slid out of the tankini, called the doctor, and decided to have the distorted and incorrect veins removed.*

I've had liposuction twice. The first time, it was on my thighs, in the saddle-bag area. This was eons ago, when liposuction was brand-new, and women were willing to trade their firstborn children to try it. Back then, we didn't know the downsides about lipo: that you can't take too much fat at once, or the blood loss could bring on a heart attack.

So I went in, had my thighs vacuumed, and thank God, it worked, in that it took away the fat from my legs. But six months later, I developed funny lumps around my waist. No one in those days knew that could happen.

When you do liposuction, you really have to commit to keeping your weight down, otherwise it comes back in weird places, in strange ways.

The best lipo procedures I've seen on anyone are under the chin on women who are born with necks that go right into their chests. Neck lipo can make a huge difference even though so little fat is taken out.

I didn't try lipo again until a few months ago, when I decided to have my upper arms done. I was especially motivated to get rid of new pockets of grandma flab that had formed around my elbow in the back. Couldn't wear short-sleeved shirts or sleeveless dresses. A terrific doctor named Lisa Cassileth did it for me.

If you are in your seventies and have a body part lipo'ed without a skin lift, be prepared to be scared to death of the result. Mine worked. My arms looked skinny, and that was great. They weren't flabby at all, but they were still wrinkled. So the next step was a minor pull-up in my armpits. This lift left small scars, but my arms, for my age, look just fine, and I don't have to go swimming in a blouse.

What's driven me to have both my legs and my arms attended to is the beauty ideal of the long, lean-limbed woman. It's a fairly recent development, this obsession with slender stems. In the nineteenth century, plump arms and chubby legs were considered delectable and precious. Now, they're considered a disgrace.

I think the giraffe aesthetic started in the Fifties, when Grace Kelly and Audrey Hepburn became the most envied actresses on screen. It was the era of models turning into actresses. Real actresses just couldn't compete. Rita Hayworth was slim, but she had some meat on her bones. Marilyn Monroe was a hog in comparison to Audrey Hepburn, as were Jayne Mansfield and Jane Russell. They were voluptuous, large-boned beauties, even in their day. In ours, they'd be playing the fat girl/best friend parts in movies . . . or providing the voices of animated hippopotami in the latest Disney film.

Normal women who would dream of comparing their gams to Cameron Diaz's—and who'd dare, really?—aren't grasping to achieve a beauty ideal. Your limbs are only as long as they are already. The under-six-feet crowd (i.e., 99 percent of human females) know they can't do anything about their height. But they can do something to make their limbs lithe, and appear taller, in the process.

## The Right to Bare Arms

So many women walk around self-conscious about their upper arms. "Hadassah hunks," by the way, is my official medical term to describe the fat and skin that hang from your upper arm. All of us have a memory of a grandma in a sleeveless dress with big, fat arms. Once you hit sixty, the skin gets so loose that normal sleeve sizes don't fit. When you do wear arm-showing clothes, you feel exposed and embarrassed if you—God forbid—have to wave at anyone or raise your hand to signal the waiter. Big arms that flap like you're about to take flight, or suffocate someone in a clench, aren't attractive or feminine.

Men have big arms. They call them "guns." Women with "guns" want to shoot themselves.

If you're under thirty-five and have fat arms and resilient skin, you'd be better off with arm lipo than a lift. It's less expensive, and you'll have no visible scars. Arm lipo, which I had, takes an hour under local anesthesia and sedation. You'll go in and get drugged and numbed. The doctor will make small incisions in your armpit to insert a small cannula—a metal tube—to infuse the area with a tumescent solution of lidocaine (a painkiller), saline, and epinephrine (to constrict blood vessels).

Once your arm is pumped up with fluid, the doctor then inserts another cannula, which is hooked up to a suction machine, and proceeds to hoover out the saline solution as well as the fat. Then your incision will be closed with a stitch or two. And you're done.

You'll have some swelling and bruising to deal with for a couple of weeks, decreasingly so. You'll also have to wear a compression sleeve on each arm for a week to hold off the worst of the swelling and to help contour your new arms.

**Pain?** Some, for a couple of days, easily held at bay by medication. When the compression garments come off, so will the sleeves of your dresses and shirts. The only scars are teeny and in your armpit. No one will ever see them. Arm lipo is relatively inexpensive. Expect to pay between $2,000 and $3,000.

The over-thirty-five-year-olds who have loose hanging skin due to the demands of gravity, age-related skin laxity, and/or the stretching out of having gained and lost a lot of weight need an arm lift, also called brachioplasty. Fourteen thousand had this done in 2007.

As most doctors explain it, the arm lift trades one aesthetic problem for another. The first problem is "bat wings." The second problem is significant, permanent scars either on the inside of the arm, from pit to elbow, or on the outside, like a seam, also from pit to elbow. A mini-brachioplasty scar is just a semi-circular crescent that spans the armpit.

The choice is yours. Big arms or big scars? If you decide to go for it and live with scars, the procedure is described below.

For an arm lift, you'll have either general anesthesia or local numbing with sedation. Whenever possible, take the local and sedation, just to avoid the scary risks of being put under. It's not like you're going to be watching the doctor slice into you. If you don't have to see it, and you won't feel it, you might as well be awake, and enjoy the Valium for the hour or two of the procedure.

The doctor will make the incision—depending on the state of your arm, it'll be on the inside, along the outside, or across the armpit. Once the incision is made, the doctor may use sutures to stitch the arm muscles tighter so your arms will be firmer and more toned-looking.

Then, if liposuction is also called for, he'll do that next, removing excess fat.

Last, he'll pull the skin around the arm tighter—not too tight, or you won't have a full range of motion—trim the excess skin, and sew the remaining skin envelope closed. Those lucky enough to get by with a mini brachioplasty will only have their skin yanked tighter toward the armpit, like tugging up your sleeve. A smaller flap of skin will be excised.

With either a full or a mini, you might have a drainage tube put in, which will come out in a few days. You'll be bandaged, and put in a compression sleeve for support and to prevent swelling.

Then the surgeon will do the whole thing all over again, on the other side.

**Drawbacks?** You'll **bruise** and **swell**, but only for a couple of weeks. You'll have **pain** for several days, but again, drugs will hold that at bay.

Whenever you're cut with a scalpel, you run the risk of **infection,** but you'll probably be on antibiotics before and after surgery to prevent it.

There's also the risk of **bleeding** from a nicked vessel, but this usually resolves itself or is corrected by your doctor fairly easily. Once the swelling is completely gone in a few months, you might notice that one arm is slightly bigger than the other.

**Asymmetry** does happen in surgery, as in nature. If anyone notices the difference, just tell them you punch harder with the bigger arm.

The major drawback is if you have the full brachioplasty, there will be **scars** running the length of your upper arm.

**Reasons to be cheerful?** Brachioplasty is considered a low-risk surgery. If you have local anesthesia, it's unlikely anything will go wrong. Plus, you'll get the arms of your dreams.

You won't be afraid to **hug a child,** for fear of crushing her.

You can **hail a taxi** and not slap the guy standing next to you with your flab.

You can **put on a tank top** when it's hot, just like everyone else.

You can wear **clothes that fit your arms *and* your torso.**

Most important, **you won't be self-conscious anymore.** You can swing your arms freely as you walk, fling them around your beloved's shoulders, arrange them akimbo on your hips, and know that, **in any position or posture, your arms look good.**

You can be miserable your whole life and do nothing. Or, you can do something, be miserable for a week, and then be happy for the rest of your life. Hardly seems a choice. All this freedom can be yours for only $5,000. A bargain, in my book.

## The Right to Bare Thighs, Too

In an hourglass figure, you don't want *all* the sand to be on the bottom. Women with thunder thighs are self-conscious about rolling down the street with them. Often, the large-legged have normal-sized or petite waists and they have to buy pants that are tight in the thighs and gigantic around the middle. It's as if they were made of halves of two different women. In photos from the waist up, they appear model-thin, or totally average-sized. But when the camera pulls back and reveals their lower half, the photographer has to attach the wide-angle lens.

A bottom half that's out of proportion to the top couldn't be more frustrating. The thigh anxiety goes way beyond having to sneak mismatched bikini tops and bottoms past the checkout girl at Bloomingdale's. You're self-conscious and fraught with fear about what heavy thighs look like, and what they might do. Every step you take, every chair you break, every orgasm you fake, you'll be cursing them.

Men might say they like meat on a woman's bones, but they don't mean the meat of an entire brontosaurus.

The only real way to reduce upper leg volume is with thighplasty, or thigh lift, which nine thousand women got in 2007.

The thigh lift is the surgical equivalent of pulling down a fat pant leg and pulling up a skinny one. It's a bit more complicated, as I'll get to in a moment. The first step on the path to slenderizing your thighs is unconsciousness. Unlike an arm lift, the thighplasty calls for cutting in a sensitive area—the groin—and I personally would not want to be awake for that. Some doctors offer local anesthesia and sedation. If you're strong-willed, take it. If you're at all wigged-out by the idea of cutting near your privates, go for general anesthesia, even though, as always, if you go under, there's a minuscule chance you won't wake up.

Once you're numb/sedated or asleep, the doctor will clean the area and make his incision. If the problem is inner-thigh jiggle, you'll need a standard or medial lift, which helps tighten the inside, front, and back of the thigh. The cut is along the bikini-line crease, starting in the front and moving all the way back to the butt. Sometimes, another incision is made, creating a V-shaped wedge of skin, which will also be removed along the inside of the thigh, groin to above the knee, so the skin envelope, when it's sewn back together, will be nice and tight (but not so tight you can't walk, run, sit, do a split, hang from a chandelier during sex, etc.).

If your complaint is saddlebags along the outer thigh, the incision will run from the bikini crease upward, across the hip at the lower panty line, and extend down to the butt crease. It's a long cut. The promise is that the scar will be hidden by underwear and bathing suits. The scar is yours to keep, but it'll fade. As with the arm lift, and the tummy tuck, for that matter, you have to decide which you hate more: the body part or the scars.

Thighplasty is often combined with liposuction of the area. Depending on your doctor's style, he'll do that before or after the incisions are made. Next, he'll pull the skin back in place, excise or remove the excess, and stitch you back together. If you had the wedge cut, you'll have a new vertical seam along the inside of your thigh from knee to crotch, as well as the curved scar along the bikini crease. You'll probably also have a drainage tube to siphon off excess fluid. That will come out in a few days. Also, you'll be cleaned, bandaged, and fit into a compression garment to stem swelling. Next, the surgeon will start all over again, on the other leg. The operation(s) will take two to four hours.

**Drawbacks?** Starting with the worst, if you had general anesthesia, there's the tiny risk of **death** on the table. Highly unlikely. Extremely remote. But, as always, I'd be remiss not to mention it at all.

Next, you've got the four constant risks of any surgery: **swelling, bruising, bleeding, pain.** All of these are temporary, preventable with medication, or easily fixable by your doctor.

The other routine risk with surgery is **infection.** I call special attention to infection with an inner thigh or medial lift because the incision is dangerously close to where you pee and poop. You have to be extremely careful not to let any urine or feces get near the wound as it heals. But even the most anally retentive can't stop every single microscopic contamination. You will need to buy a large bottle of antibiotic soap and wash in the shower after every trip to the toilet.

Some doctors close this wound with Dermabond, a medical Krazy Glue, to seal the area to better prevent infection. California surgeon Dr. Lisa Cassileth told me her infection rate went from 70 percent down to five percent by covering the incision with Dermabond. It'll peel off on its own after a few weeks, around the time the wound is healed.

You **can't have sex** until the three-week mark.*

**Asymmetry** is also a worry. But if both your legs are smaller, does it really matter if one is slightly smaller than the other? If the difference is freakish, complain to your surgeon and get a follow-up lipo to even them out. Also, you might have numb spots from nerve damage, which will most likely wear off in a few months.

**The benefits? No more skirt-style bathing suit bottoms or sarongs across your hips at the beach.**

You can **wear jeans.** Not fat-girl jeans, either. Skinny jeans!

Also, you can't exert yourself for two months. **Slack off and enjoy it.** All the time you'd spend at the gym to get rid of those thighs? You can spend it now doing whatever unhealthy activity you choose (except smoking, which interferes with healing).

And when you do go back to the gym, and your thighs are half as big as they were, won't you **shock and amaze everyone** there! You will have to wait six weeks for the wounds to heal, but it'll be worth the wait and the $4,000 to $7,500 you'll pay for the thighplasty.

# You're So Vein, You Probably Think This Section Is About You

Do your legs look like a road map of Russia? Lots of swollen, snaking red and blue varicose and spider veins? Why you have them, not

---

*But you can always tell your husband it could be up to a year, if he no longer turns you on.

even the smartest doctor can say. Blame your parents, of course. You blame them for everything else, and visible veins are genetically inherited.

Also, you might have a job that has you standing a lot.

Or sitting a lot.

Maybe you exercise too much.

Or too little.

The only thing we know for sure: the valves in your leg veins are not doing their job right, and, as a result, blood gets re-routed into venous dead ends that twist, turn, bulge under the skin, or turn into branched reservoirs that look vaguely like webs. "Web veins" sound slightly more appealing than "spider veins." Doesn't matter. You could call them Gisele Bündchen, and they'd still be ugly. Besides making you look ancient, varicose and spider veins can swell, ache, bleed, and cause ulcers on your legs.

Here are three options to get rid of the squiggles, in descending order of magnitude:

## Vein Ligation and Stripping

This procedure is for large, close-to-the-surface saphenous veins. It's the most drastic option and the most painful. The operation, which you can have under general anesthesia if you prefer, is considered minor. The doctor makes an incision or cut at the top of the vein in the groin area. It's tied, or ligated, to stop blood flow. Then a second cut is made at the bottom of the vein by the ankle. A thin wire is threaded from the ankle incision up the vein to the groin. And then the wire is pulled out, bringing the vein and all its branches along with it.

The one mitigating factor about removing the saphenous vein? It's what cardiac surgeons use for heart-bypass operations. If you have your leg vein stripped, you'd better take care of your heart!

The soft-core version of vein stripping is called ambulatory

phlebectomy, a similar process that surgically removes smaller varicose veins, one at a time. With this, you need only local anesthesia.

A friend of mine had her veins stripped a few years ago. At the
time, she was thirty-eight, thin and gorgeous, but was absolutely obsessed with her wormy-looking legs. She said the procedure itself
didn't hurt (she was knocked out), but for days afterward, she had
throbbing pain in both legs and hated the compression garments she
had to wear for two weeks. A good patient, she followed doctor's orders about taking ten short walks a day, and keeping her legs elevated
otherwise, and ended up thrilled with the results: her legs are smooth
and pink, and look like they belong on her young body, and not on
her eighty-year-old grandmother's.

The procedure takes one to four hours, depending on how bad
your veins are. It'll cost between $1,000 and $3,000 per leg. There's
always the risk that more varicose veins will develop. In up to 90 percent of cases, your legs will stay vein-free forever.

## Sclerotherapy

This is a very popular (384,000 had it in 2007) no-knives treatment
for small varicose veins. The doctor fills a syringe with a mixture of a
painkiller and a sclerosing agent (either a saline or an alcohol-based
solution) and then injects it directly into the varicose vein. The sclerosing agent irritates the walls of the veins, causing them to collapse.
Collapsed veins mean no blood can get into them, rendering them
invisible on the surface of your skin.

Eventually, the out-of-commission vein is absorbed by the body.
You might have some redness on your leg afterwards or bruising.
You'll also have to wear compression garments and take short walks
many times a day. No downtime here, you can resume lunching and
shopping immediately.

The length of the procedure is one to two hours and costs between

$150 and $500 per leg, per treatment. The risks are few: discoloration around the injection sites, which might take a few months to fade, a possible and rare blood clot might form where the vein used to be, the possibility of an allergic reaction, some swelling, bruising, and minimal, manageable pain.

In an odd complication, you can't take birth-control pills for six weeks before and six weeks after sclerotherapy, due to the risk of hemorrhaging. It'd be horrible to have sclerotherapy to remove veins, go off the pill, get knocked up by mistake/accident, and then get a huge new crop of varicose veins during pregnancy, that need to be treated with sclerotherapy, so you go off the pill . . . and so on.

Before you know it, you'll have more kids than veins.

## Laser Vein Treatment

This is for spider veins, the web-like matrix of red veins that are under the surface of the legs. To start a treatment, the doctor will apply a clear, cool lubricant to your legs to protect the surface skin from the laser. Then he'll zap you in the spider veins with a hand-held device.

The laser feels a bit like a snap on your flesh, but it doesn't hurt enough to get sedation or even topical numbing. The laser penetrates the skin layers and is absorbed by the vein's red pigments. The hemoglobin can't take the laser heat and coagulates. The vein can't take the clotting pressure, so it collapses.

Again, eventually, your body will absorb the spent veins.

The whole procedure takes less than an hour. You can return to your life, already in progress, as soon as you leave the doctor's office. You might be a little red, but not so you or anyone else would care.

The one catch about laser treatments: you can't get results after just one session. You'll need to go back every six weeks for four or five sessions. But at the end of the six-month course of treatment and the $2,000 or so you'll spend, the spider veins will be eighty percent gone. And good riddance.

# Hands and Feet

Have you seen Madonna's hands lately? She's got the face of a thirty-year-old, the body of a twenty-year-old, and the hands of an eighty-year-old crone. Hands are an easy giveaway of a woman's age.* Fortunately, there're a lot of procedures to make them look as young as the rest of you.

## Hands

The reason hands are so hard-hit by aging is exposure. Many women are very good about putting sunscreen on their faces every day, but how many of us remember to put it on the back of our hands? The sun saps collagen and elastin, making skin lax, and causes pigmentation problems, aka dark spots. Plunging our hands into hot water to wash dishes sucks the moisture out of our skin, which speeds collagen and elastic erosion. What's more, as we age, we lose fat on the hands, making all the bones and veins more obvious.

So what to do? First matter of business: re-plump the hands to hide the bones and veins. You can refill bony areas with a fat transfer, taking adipose tissue from where you don't need it (hips, belly, butt) and injecting purified cells under the skin of your hands. The fat cells that create new blood-supply connections—about half—will take up permanent residence in your hands. The rest will be absorbed by your body, which is why doctors tend to overfill.

The alternative to a fat transfer is refilling bony hands with a hyaluronic filler like Restylane, Juvéderm Ultra, or Perlane. The process is simple. You'll get injections under the skin at the doctor's office, and the effects will last up to eight months, depending on which filler your doctor recommends. In terms of cost efficiency, a fat transfer is more expensive, but it's a one-time fee. Fillers are less

*Except for the Venus de Milo, lucky bitch.

pricey, but you'll have to get injections repeatedly to maintain the results.

Once your hands are plumped up, you can firm up the skin via laser resurfacing. A fractionated laser resurfacing involves the surgeon zapping your skin with the hand-held laser wand. The heat from the laser penetrates deep into the dermal layer of skin, stimulating new growth of firming collagen and elastin. The results will become evident in a month and increasingly so over the next six months.

Finally, for the complete hand rejuvenation, you'll have to remove the age spots. A pigmented laser can take care of those. The doctor will zap them with the laser several times, and the spot will peel away.

A full hand job—including fat transfer or filler, resurfacing, and spot removal—costs between $5,000 and $8,000.

## Feet

Although feet do get bonier with age, the change isn't obvious, thanks to the fact that *we wear shoes all day long, hello!*

However, standing and walking for decades worsens bunions. Bunion removal surgery is extremely complicated. In fact, there are a hundred different ways to do it, depending on the individual case. That said, all of the procedures involve bone, ligament, and tendon removal. Full recovery takes at least eight weeks and up to six months. Immediately after surgery, you have to stay off the foot for a couple of weeks. The pins and stitches will come out within a month. You'll have to wear a walking cast or special shoes for two months and resume normal activities at that time.

Bunion surgery costs anywhere from $3,000 to $10,000, but it will be, at least partially, covered by medical insurance.

Be very careful about this one. According to studies, up to 33 percent of people who had bunion surgery weren't happy with the result. Most doctors warn against any elective foot surgery.

Unless the bunions are so painful that every step hurts, don't do it.

God forbid something goes wrong, and you can't walk again. Or you lose a digit. A friend of a friend went in to have her bunion removed, and, during the recovery period, her big toe got gangrene and half of it had to be cut off.

She'll never wear flip-flops again.

Some women voluntarily had their toes lopped off. I remember reading in Alex Kuczynski's book *Beauty Junkies* about a woman who had her toes shortened to fit into Jimmy Choo shoes. Okay, that's insane!

She'll never play "This Little Piggy Went to Market" again.

But at least she gets 10 percent off on a pedicure.

## Shrinking the Birthday Suit After Massive Weight Loss

Attention contestants on "The Biggest Loser." After a massive weight loss of a hundred or more pounds, even more resilient skin can only bounce back so much. The skin had been stretched and thinned so much, it hangs over a newly slimmed body like a rubber suit. Fortunately, a plastic surgeon can help to resize the suit via a series of lifts on the lower body, back, arms, breasts, face, and neck.

**Lower body lift or belt lipectomy.** The patient is given general anesthesia. Then, the surgeon makes a large incision all the way around the body—hence "belt"—at the top of the bikini line. "If the whole butt, thighs, mons area, tummy in front and lower back are sagging and have hanging skin, a lower body lift is appropriate," said California surgeon and friend Dr. Lisa Cassileth. "It's essentially like pulling up a new pair of pants." Once the incision is made, the doctor does just that, hoisting up the skin in the outer thighs and butt and pulling down the tummy and lower back, excising the excess panniculus adiposus (or folds of skin), and sewing back together what remains. The scar will encircle the waist. It's permanent but will fade over time.

**Inner thigh lift.** A belt lipectomy will take care of the outer thighs but not the inside. To take up the slack on the inner thighs, the patient is put to sleep, and the surgeon makes an incision in the crease where thigh meets crotch, front to back. A V-shaped wedge on the inner thigh might also be necessary. The skin is lifted, excess is removed, and the incisions are closed. The scars are also permanent but will fade.

**Upper back lift.** The lower body lift attends to the rolls of skin on the lower back. But often, there are also rolls hanging from the mid-back area, too. The incisions in this case start at the mid-spine and sweep downward following the curve of the shoulder blades on each side. The scar will look like an upside-down V. The excess rolls are gathered and excised, and the remaining skin is sutured closed.

**Arm lift.** A standard brachioplasty to remove hanging skin on the upper arms might not be enough. So, instead of making an incision in the armpit or the length of the arm from pit to elbow, the surgeon will do *both*. "It's a T-shaped incision," said Dr. Cassileth—the short stroke across the armpit and the long one down to the elbow. Same drill: the sags are lifted, extra skin is removed, and the incisions are closed tighter. Also, with body lifts, the scars are permanent but they'll fade over time.

**Breast lift.** Again, a standard "anchor" lift might not be enough for women who've had massive weight loss. The problem is their stretched-out skin can't support the new breast placement. "I take the skin you'd normally throw away, create an internal bra to support the lifted breast with it, and then drape the outer skin envelope on top. It's a double layer of skin for extra support to ensure that the breast won't droop three months later." The outer suturing looks the same, the classic anchor-shaped scar.

**Face/Neck Lift.** The usual lift incisions for face and neck—under the chin, in front of and behind the ears—should be enough to address the hanging skin in that area. If not, the surgeon can also make an incision in the back of the neck, behind the hairline where the scalp meets the neck, to deal with any extra skin that might be back there. The surgeon will do the usual lifting of skin, excising the folds, and closing the incisions.

Recovery for all lifts includes the usual problems of swelling, bruising, risk of infection, pain, scars, and bleeding. Although a few surgeries can be done at a time, you can't possibly do them all in one shot. You'll have to have multiple operations over the course of six months to a year. Also, expect to pay a fortune to get rid of that excess skin. Insurance won't cover these operations, and, all added up, the total might be what you make in a year. Or more. BUT—once you get rid of all that skin that's weighing you down, you'll look so great, you'll be able to go get a better job that pays more. Consider body contouring after major weight loss an investment in your svelte future.

$$\left(\;\textbf{Fourteen}\;\right)$$

# **Vaginas** and **Butts**

*Joan was beginning to really look like a swan—she was metamorphosing into the beauty she had always been on the inside. There would be no end to what she could accomplish once she had reached her full potential. Joan was beginning to get excited, but her work had not yet ended. She knew she had to continue to be honest with herself, and speaking of ends, hers was a mess! Joan knew her flat ass was to asses as Yoko Ono's singing voice was to the sounds of cats mating while trapped in a bag.*

*Thanks to J.Lo, Joan knew that men liked a round bootylicious butt, and she decided that she would do anything to get one as she NEEDED to be "Joanie from the Block."*

*She had been invited to a big birthday party that night by her Barbie neighbor next door and was being fixed up with a single straight guy, with a job. Joan knew she didn't have time to get padding, so she rushed to a party supply store and bought two helium-filled Mylar balloons. She carefully shoved them into her bloomers and arrived at the party with a butt that, well, kicked ass!*

*Her blind date could not stop staring at Joan's round bottom and she was thrilled as she knew this time she was making herself beautiful on her own without help from a doctor or a needle. Joan was beaming, until dinner was served. She had not factored in how dangerous it might be to sit down.*

*Halfway through the appetizer, the Mylar balloons released a double-barreled stereo fart, the likes of which had not been heard since Guinness inducted the world's largest whoopee cushion into its annals. Joan was mortified. She excused herself, making up some crazy story about forgetting to take her Beano. Needless to say, she was defeated and deflated. Her date left with someone else, and Joan met with a plastic surgeon the next day to get exactly what she felt like—an ass. The cute young doctor (single, straight, and Jewish, incidentally) was instantly smitten with Joan, and she felt the same attraction towards him . . .*

"You're right. Men do like big boobs," said David Matlock, a board-certified gynecological surgeon. "But they also like a tight vagina."

Dr. Matlock, who is the trademark holder for the phrases "Laser Vaginal Rejuvenation," "Designer Laser Vaginoplasty," "G-Spot Amplification," and "G-Shot," does hundreds of surgeries every year on women's private parts in his Los Angeles surgical practice, so he should know.

Is this cosmetic surgery's final frontier? The va-jay-jay is getting lifted, tucked, and resurfaced. Although fewer than 1,500 women and a smattering of transsexuals had vaginoplasty in 2007, the procedure is getting more popular. In Los Angeles, everyone's talking about it. They're not all putting their money where their genitals are—yet. But it seems inevitable that down-under beauty has come of age.

When the baby boomers get as old as I am, they will learn the hideous truth that I wish my mother had warned me about: one day, your vagina will fall out. It's just like how men's balls drop, and they can start playing golf with them.

I woke up a few months ago, and I thought, Why am I wearing a bunny slipper? And why is it gray? Then I realized, That's my vagina!

It can be a good thing, though. When you get a hot flash, you can wipe your forehead with your vagina. When you're sixty, you can have sex in the bedroom and watch TV in the living room—at the same time. If these prospects don't appeal to you, however, you can have your vagina retooled. And I don't mean by the hunky handyman.

Plastic surgeons offer a procedure to tighten the nether regions to make you like a virgin, which I'll describe in minute detail. Or, you can have yourself sewn back together so that your vagina stays inside you, where your husband can find it. Otherwise, it's like he's lost the keys again. Honestly, no one wants to be in bed and hear her husband ask, "Honey, have you seen your vagina? I can't find it anywhere. I looked in all the usual places."

Ten years ago, who'd have thought that women would care about the appearance of their bits and pieces? Until now, that area was the only part of a woman's body we *weren't* self-conscious about. Men, on the other hand, have always been anxiety-ridden about their penises, ever since the first cavewoman asked, "Is it in yet?"

The days of carefree disregard for our vulvas and vaginas are officially over. A critic would say that the doctors who invented these procedures were digging deep into women's bottomless pit of insecurity. And that critic would be right!

You could also blame Internet pornography. A new generation of men has gotten so used to the vaginas they see on screen that they have no idea what real ones look like.* Porn stars were some of the first to get their vaginas fixed. Adult film mega-star Jenna Jameson, author of *How to Make Love Like a Porn Star*, had her bits overhauled (allegedly). And, as reported at gossip sites, she's not happy about it. I read she's holed up (as it were) until she can get herself re-done.

---

*And unless they back away from their computers, they never will.

Like most cosmetic surgeries, the goal of a vagina lift is to make the woman look refreshed, tighter, and younger. Unfortunately, your vagina has one sign of its true age, no matter what you do to it.

Most people don't know this, but a man can tell a woman's age by counting the rings in her uterus. To do so, however, he needs a flashlight. And a miner's hat. If you make love in the dark, though, your vagina will be only as old as it looks.

As well as aesthetic enhancement, vaginal renovation tightens the area, too. Roseanne Barr said she got a vaginal rejuvenation, and now she's got "a va-junior."

The vaginal muscles get stretched out from childbirth. Vaginal rejuvenation can help. The goal is to shrink the circumference of the interior vagina. To make the tunnel a tighter squeeze, for greater erotic pleasure during intercourse. Also, vaginal tightening improves bladder control and can reduce vaginal farting.*

Other down-under procedures trim the lips for a neater appearance, add or decrease volume to the pudenda, and even restore virginity!

I'm not sure how I feel about women taking lasers to their genitals to look like porn stars. But if you're preoccupied by the appearance of your vulva, or if you have an abnormality that causes pain or chafing, or are completely loose inside from delivering nine-pound babies, then get to the seat of the problem and consider surgical/vaginal intervention.

I asked Dr. Matlock to explain the latest procedures being done in this field, including:

## Vaginal Rejuvenation

To tighten a vagina that's been loosened by childbirth and aging, you can have the tunnel narrowed to your specifications (one-finger, two-

*My cousin Edie's farts were so loud, her gynecologist wore earplugs.

finger, etc.). "Women say, 'I want to be sixteen again,' " he said. "It's all about increasing friction. The problem my patients have is vaginal relaxation, from childbirth usually. I go in, take the laser, open up the lining of the vagina, tighten the muscles with suture material on the top, bottom, and inside, to decrease the diameter. And we make them look pretty at the same time."

He said 98 percent of his patients opt for general anesthesia, along with a pudendal block that keeps their insides numb for eighteen to twenty-four hours. When that wears off, the level of pain is similar to recovering from an episiotomy. The patient can go back to work in seven days, and have sex again in six weeks.

**Risks:** Like any surgery, be wary of bleeding and infection. The chances are less than one percent, but you might end up with hypo-sensation, or hypersensation (too little feeling or too much). In some cases, women ask for a vagina that turns out to be *too* tight. The surgeon can fix that in quick follow-up surgery.

**Rewards:** Enhanced sexual gratification. Yes, for your husband. For you? Maybe.

**$$$$:** $9,000 to $10,800.

## Reduction Labioplasty

To reduce the labia minora (the inner lips) that protrude too far out of the labia majora (the outer lips), the doctor will use a laser for trimming and suture for closing the wounds. Having extensive labia minora overhang can cause pain and chafing while playing sports as well as during sex. Doctors use a laser to make the incisions, cutting in a semicircular contour to get rid of the slack labia minora, and then stitching it up with dissolving sutures. Most women choose local numbing and sedation, or twilight anesthesia, where you're half asleep. You'll be back at work in seven days, back in the saddle in six weeks.

**Risks:** Same as above. Bleeding, infection. Loss of sensation or possibly too much feeling. The side effects are rare.

**Rewards:** You can wear sexy underwear without worrying that your lips are showing. And save a fortune on Chapstick. You can go running without injuring your parts.

$$$: $8,000 to $9,000.

## Augmentation Labioplasty

The labia majora, or outer lips, thin with age. Just another place where you have age-related fat loss in another place you'd like to keep it. To plump up the labia majora for a younger-looking vulva, your best option is a fat transfer. The doctor sucks the fat out of you where you don't need it, treats it to prepare it for transfer, and then injects the purified adipose into your outer vaginal lips. If the cells can form a new blood supply, they'll nestle into their new home happily. Otherwise, they'll be absorbed by the body. Expect to keep about half of the fat transferred.

For this reason, often doctors will overfill the transfer area. Expect to spend a few days off your feet with your legs spread wide open before you can close them comfortably. You'll want serious local anesthesia in both areas, the place where you harvest the fat and where you transfer it to, as well as sedation. Since there are no open wounds to heal and the incisions are so small you don't need stitches, you'll be back at work the next day, back to sex in a week.

**Risks:** The usual. Bleeding and infection. Otherwise, the chance that the fat won't stick, and you'll have to do it again.

**Rewards:** Purely cosmetic.

$$: $5,000

## Clitoral Prepuce Reduction

For aesthetic or erotic reasons, some women want the flap of skin that covers the clitoris—the prepuce—reduced and to have a thin membrane that's draped prettily over the clitoris. Doctors liken this aesthetic procedure to a circumcision, the reduction of the female version of a foreskin—not to be confused with the horrible mutilation done to women in Africa. It's done under local or general, whichever his patient wants. She'll be back at work in a week, can have sex again in six weeks.

**Risks:** Bleeding, infection. Loss of sensation or too much sensation.

**Rewards:** It looks nicer, the clitoris is easier to find, and sensation might be accentuated.

**$$$:** $8,000 to $9,000

## Perineoplasty

To tighten the area of skin between the vagina and the anus. The perineum is where the introitus muscles are located—the ones that keep the vaginal opening narrow. If you have a large opening, this procedure can narrow it. Another procedure that's all about using a laser to make incisions, and then the surgeon stitches everything tighter with dissolving sutures. You can have sedation and local numbing or general anesthesia. You'll be right as rain for work in a week and can road-test the new vaginal opening in six weeks.

**Risks:** Mainly infection and bleeding.

**Rewards:** A smaller opening. Good sexually for both of you.

**$$$:** $6,000 to $8,000

## Hymen Restoration

Yes, Virginia, you *can* have your hymen reattached and be a virgin all over again. Apparently, Middle Eastern women who go to college in America have their fun and then return to Egypt and Saudi Arabia for their arranged marriages to men who demand virgin brides, can get a potentially lifesaving hymenoplasty.

If you've had children—via vaginal delivery—the scraps of your hymen are beyond restoration, so forget it. Those who haven't given birth yet can undergo this procedure, which is done under local anesthesia. It's a bit like fixing a torn earlobe. When the hymen, a thin membrane about a third of the way in the vagina, is broken, it doesn't disappear. The torn parts remain in place. To re-fuse them together, the doctor has to re-open the skin, "de-nude" it, to create an open wound. He'll stitch two open parts together, and, during healing, they'll reconnect. When the patient has sex again, the man will feel resistance, and she'll bleed a bit when the restored hymen tears.

**Risks:** Infection, bleeding, but so minimal it's almost not worth mentioning.

**Rewards:** Not being killed on your wedding night.

**$$:** $2,400 to $5,000

## Vulva Lipoplasty

If you think you've got a fat vagina, this is for you. Incredibly, this procedure is billed to treat women who have unsightly fat bulges in their vulva.* It's a small lipo procedure, done wherever you have fat deposits on the pubic mound or the lips.

"It's liposculpting," said Dr. Matlock. "Women want to get rid of the fat that sags into the upper half of the labia majora. A nineteen-year-old ballerina came in and said she was self-conscious in her tutu. It showed too much, looked puffy." So, she had her vulva suctioned to be as skinny as the rest of her. A micro-cannula is put in the fatty area, and the excess adipose is sucked out. You'll want local numbing and sedation for this.

---

*Since most women don't walk around flashing their genitalia, the first question that jumped to my mind was "Unsightly *to whom?*" Perhaps your husband recently said to you, "When you gain weight, it really shows in your vagina." Or some cruel kids in the neighborhood called you a "fat vulva" when you walked by on the street. If you can stand to lose a few around the vagina, pay attention.

**Risks:** Infection, bleeding, bruising, swelling. Just like any lipo procedure, you might have bumps.

**Rewards:** After you've been reduced, don't expect people to come up to you at parties and say, "Have you lost weight? What's your secret?" But you'll look less rounded in panties and bathing suits. Without too much fat cushion, you might feel more sensation during intercourse.

**$$$:** $6,000 to $8,000

## G-spot Amplification

Another brand new "lunchtime procedure," this procedure is quick and easy. The doctor will give you a shot of local anesthetic, and then he'll inject human-derived collagen into the G-spot area on the anterior wall of your vagina. You have to wear a tampon for several hours.* The results will last four months, until the collagen is absorbed by your body. Ideally, a plumped up G-spot will mean added erotic intensity, loads more fun in bed. The procedure takes half an hour. There was a study that claimed 87 percent of women reported enhanced sexual arousal and gratification from this procedure. You can go back to work immediately.

**Risks:** None. No allergic reaction to collagen. No cutting, and therefore you're safe from infection and bleeding.

**Rewards:** Better sex. G-spot stimulation that might otherwise have been neglected.

**$$:** $1,850 for a single shot, $2,500 for double.

---

*If you're over 55, this will make you feel girlish again.

# Butt That's Not All, Folks

Why have Jennifer Lopez, Jessica Biel, and Jessica Alba risen to fame and fortune? Is it because they all have names that begin with the letter J? Is it their pretty faces? It's definitely not their acting talent.

It's because of their rears! Scarlett Johansson is a very talented actress, but her rear end emotes more depth of feeling than all of Lindsay Lohan's parts combined. There's a reason Johansson is so often filmed from behind. *Her behind!*

A high, hard ass is a thing of beauty we can all appreciate. If your booty is rounded, firm (yet pliant), and undimpled, men will form a line behind you as you walk down the street. We all know there are men who consider themselves connoisseurs of women's breasts and legs. But every man is an ass man.* This is why they might not check you out (overtly) when you're coming toward them, but they'll always turn around to check out the rear view as you walk by. They can't help themselves. When men come eye-to-cheek with a bouncy butt, they go soft in the brain.

Unfortunately, not all women were born with a million-dollar tush. The J. Lo ass is a gift from God and good genes.

That said, you *can* make improvements on the rump you've got: bigger, smaller, higher, smoother. With enough money and time, you could probably train your husband to sit up and beg!

# To Make a Butt Smaller

**Liposuction** is the number-one choice of doctors for reducing volume. For a long discussion of how liposuction is done, check out Chapter 10: Sucks to Be You: Lipo! Specifically, for the butt, the cannula incisions are made in strategic spots. To get at fat in the junction where thigh meets ass, the cannula is inserted in the crease, or the

---

*Especially the gay ones.

underside of the cheek. To get at upper-butt fat, including any hate handle action, the doctor makes the cannula incisions in the two little dimples of the lower back. Hence, all scars are well hidden by the contours of your natural anatomy. Any single lipo procedure starts at $3,000 and can go up to $7,000.

**Recovery:** You'll be sore for a few days and swollen for three weeks. You won't see the full results for up to six months, due to swelling. You'll have to wear a compression garment, like a girdle, for a month or longer. To speed healing, move around and do light activities as soon as possible. Get back to work within a week and go back to the gym in six weeks.

**Risks:** As with any lipo procedure, the main risks are swelling, pain, infection, bruising, numbness. All of the risks are temporary or can be prevented or eased with drugs.

**Rewards:** A slimmer rear, more confidence, shopping for jeans without crying, taking up only one seat on the subway.

## To Make a Butt Higher

Due to aging or significant weight loss, the skin of one's butt might become sagging and droopy. Women with old-lady asses need granny panties to accommodate all that extra flesh. Gravity has had its way with their butts. Surgery to the rescue. What we have to solve the loose caboose problem is a **butt lift.**

To lift a butt, your doctor will give you general anesthesia. It's a fairly long surgery, three to five hours. Once you're under, lying face down on the table, the doctor will clean the area and make his dotted lines with a marker. The incisions will be above the butt, in a two-humped horizontal line, from hip to hip. The incision is shaped the way artists draw flying birds in the distance. The next step is to raise the skin to a higher position over your muscle layer. Once a desired tension is reached (tight enough to look great in clingy skirts, loose enough to sit down and accommodate the fat transfer), the doctor will trim the extra skin and reconnect what's left to your lower back. The scar is permanent and long, the width of your back. It's hidden in panties and bathing suits for the most part. You can combine liposuction with a butt lift, as big-bottomed ladies often do. A butt lift costs from $6,000 to $9,000.

**Recovery:** Some pain for three days. A week before you can go back to work. A month before you sit without wincing. Three months to restart an exercise routine. Six months before all the swelling is gone.

**Risks:** The usual surgical woes, including the minuscule risk of death due to complications of general anesthesia, bruising, swelling, infection, bleeding, pain, temporary loss of sensation. In other words, nothing you can't handle, or that your doctor won't warn you about and/or help you handle with meds and great advice, which you should follow to the letter. Be prepared by purchasing an inflatable plastic doughnut to sit on for a while, as well as ice packs.

**Rewards:** Who doesn't want to make men gasp in amazement when you walk by? Or have a juicy ass to put inside your Juicy Couture track pants? Every woman wants a butt that makes men weep— with appreciation, for a change.

## To Make A Butt Bigger

Incredibly, some women need to have fat put into their rears, not taken out. To address the bony bottom, we have a **fat transfer.** If your skin is firm but the booty is flat, this procedure's for you. First, the doctor will harvest some fat from the abdomen, belly, or thighs. To do so he'll insert a cannula and flood the area with a solution of saline, epinephrine, and lidocaine to make the liposuction safer and easier on your vessels and tissue. Once he's removed adequate fat, it will be processed—separated from the saline solution and blood—to be prepared for transfer into the behind. Next, using a large syringe loaded with purified fat, the doctor will inject it into or over the gluteus-soon-to-be-maximus muscles. If you're lucky, the fat will quickly adapt to its new home, making new blood supply connections and settling in for the long haul. As usual with fat transfers, some of it— percentages range from 10 to 50 percent—will be absorbed by the body. Because of this, doctors often overfill. When he's done adding the fat, you'll be cleaned, bandaged, and put in a compression girdle. You can go home that day, with an escort, as long as you've paid the $5,000 to $10,000 bill.

Another option is rear end **implants.** Candidates for butt implants are women who don't have enough fat on their abdomen to transfer into their ass, or who don't want the two-step process of a fat transfer. Instead, they opt for having a silicone pad inserted into their butt. It's a single-process procedure, and therefore less expensive than a fat transfer.

In slang terms, this is getting a boob job for your booty.

The implants are made of soft silicone that won't leak, are FDA-approved, and come in a variety of shapes and sizes. You and your doctor can page through the catalogue, and decide whether you want a bubble butt or a saucy-sloped rear. Unlike a fat transfer, with implants, you can be precise about shape.

The surgery is very similar to a boob job. You'll be given general anesthesia. When you're asleep, the surgeon will clean the area and make a vertical incision by the tailbone, above the intragluteal crease, aka "the crack." Using a scalpel and retractor, the doctor will then tunnel into the butt and make a snug pocket for the implant. The pocket is either submuscular (under the muscle) or subfascial (under the membrane between the muscle and skin). Most rear-end implants are submuscular because they look better and more natural and are impossible to feel from the outside.

Once the pocket is ready, the implant is placed inside. The doctor makes sure it's a snug fit so it won't slide down and that the two sides are symmetrical. You don't want one cheek bigger than the other or lopsided. Then, the doctor closes the pocket with stitches, as well as the incision by the tailbone. You'll have a drainage tube, some bandaging, and a compression girdle. The tube comes out in a few days. The girdle? You'll have to wear that for a few weeks. The procedure, start to finish, is a couple of hours long, and costs $5,000 to $7,000.

**Recovery:** You'll have to sleep on your belly for a month. No sitting for a few weeks, or longer. You'll be stiff and sore for a couple of weeks while the muscles stretch around the implant. You can go back to work after two weeks; back to the gym in two months.

**Risks:** I saw a crazy video on YouTube of a woman whose implants had slipped out of the pocket and drifted down to her upper thigh. This should not happen, but, alas, it did. I can't imagine what kind of bozo did her surgery.

Check your doctor's credentials! Don't have a carpenter do your implants.

Other risks include the usual surgical issues of infection, bleeding, swelling, bruising, and pain. Nothing out of the ordinary. Most of it will be prevented or medicated.

**Rewards:** If you've always had a bony butt, implants can serve as permanent padding. Never again will you bruise yourself when you sit down on a hard chair. You won't dread stadium seating. And, with a new set of bum-flaps, your husband will fall madly in love with you all over again.

## Down Under Crunches

In the old days—the 1980s—women did Kegel crunches to tighten their vaginas without a single stitch. Nowadays, they've added using a resistance device. A popular model is the GyneFlex, a V-shaped piece of plastic which is like a tiny Thigh Master (paging Suzanne Somers) for your vagina. It costs $40. If you include vag crunches in your daily workout (I believe there is a muscle group you might've ignored at the gym), you can enhance your sexual response, stop incontinence, and strengthen your perineum for power pooping. You simply insert it, V-point in, vertically. Then you attempt to clench your vaginal muscles and make the tips of the V click together. Since my vagina fell out, I can't possibly do this. So I asked my spy to give it a go. Here's her report:

"Let me just say, abdominal crunches are nothing compared to vaginal crunches! I could more easily lift an elephant with my tongue than make the GyneFlex tips touch. When you order it from their website, they send a box with two different devices, one for beginners and one for intermediate vaginal crushers. I used the beginner's GyneFlex, and could barely budge it! My vagina is a weakling! I had no idea. I made a vow to use the GyneFlex as instructed, doing a series of crunch reps every day and night until I saw improvement. I worried that I'd stress out the muscles. How might I ice them? The prospect didn't seem all that appealing.

"I kept it up, doggedly inserting the GyneFlex and bearing down like I was trying to give birth to it. In one week, I noticed some improvement in my muscle tone. Instead of pathetic quivering mush against the plastic gizmo, my vag was able to budge it a millimeter.

"Not enough progress to stay encouraged. I gave up on the GyneFlex after a few weeks, deciding to not add any more pressure to my life unless absolutely necessary. I'll try again at some point. When I'm eighty and incontinent and don't have a choice."

( **Fifteen** )

# **Finishing** Touches

*Joan had no idea—could never have imagined in her wildest dreams—that the makeover she had embarked upon not so long ago would result in so many wonderful changes in her life. She now had a gorgeous face, a sexy body, and best of all, a diamond wedding ring the size of a small asteroid on her well-manicured finger, from her new husband—the very last doctor she met in the previous chapter. Imagine. Marrying your own plastic surgeon!*

I have a philosophy about being a celebrity. Most people get to see you once in your life. So you should look good when they see you. You'd *better* look good, because after seeing a celebrity, no one asks, "Was he or she a nice person?" or "Does he or she give to charity?" No! They ask, *"So what did he or she look like?"*

From the very beginning, I always tried to look good so no one could say, "Saw her in a restaurant eating corn—made sense since she was a pig."

My everyday beauty routine is simple. I get up, look in the mirror, have a good cry, then I exercise. Thirty minutes on the treadmill and training with free weights.

Next, Adele Fass,* my fantastic makeup artist for sixteen years, does my face. She asks two important questions: "What are you doing today?" and "What color are you wearing?" For ten years, the answer has been black. The one time she didn't ask, I wore red.

I've got makeup tips galore from Adele—I'll get to those in a second. But my point here is that every woman should start her day with the same idea: that anyone she sees, anyone she meets, will be able to report back to anyone else who might care that she looks great.

Every woman should exercise, especially older women, to maintain strength and flexibility and prevent the dreaded osteoporosis.

And every woman should take five minutes out of her morning to slap on some makeup. Very scary when I see myself without any makeup. Gives me the willies. I think, "Who is that old man?"

I'm not pretty without makeup. I was never the natural beauty. No man has ever told me that I'm beautiful. That's why I do so many procedures, the constant push to look my best. I do think everyone should do whatever she can to look as good as she can.

My mother's dying words were, "Look good at my funeral. There'll be a lot of relatives there. You can cry at home." At this point in my life, I just feel better with makeup on. Everyone wants to look good— and good means groomed, pulled together, elegant.

When I go out without makeup, the doorman pukes on the welcome mat.

I don't believe makeup should be optional after age thirty-five. You owe it to yourself and to anyone who looks at you to clean yourself up, put on the finishing touches, and dress nicely. The people you see will appreciate it. And, truly, you'll feel more confident all day

---

*Adele is a makeup artist to the greats, the near-greats, the would-be greats, and a lot of rich second wives.

long, too. Now that you have a rejuvenated face, don't give it short shrift.

Polish the diamond!

Following are some finishing touches ideas to keep in mind as you proceed in your new life and new nose/tummy/face:

**Moisturize.** You should use moisturizer every day. Adele recommends an SPF of at least 15. And you should remoisturize as needed during the day. "If you're wearing makeup and you start to crack, you can remoisturize by patting or pressing it into your skin. It won't melt the makeup and makes you look fresh."

**Exfoliate.** Once a week. "Give your skin a good scrub with an exfoliating cleanser. I like apricot," said Adele. "Also, in an ideal world, you should get a facial once a month to exfoliate and clean your pores."

Some facials do a better job of that than others. A good, old-fashioned extraction facial gets rid of blackheads and rehydrates the skin. But this is 2009, and technology has advanced beyond pinching with rubber gloves. Some of the methods are bull. Oxygen facials? Please! No doctor alive will say this actually hydrates or improves the quality of your skin. You might as well push your dog aside and stick your head out the car window when driving.

One treatment that actually works—according to the studies I read—is the blue-light facial. The high-intensity blue light kills the bacteria P. acnes, which clogs pores and causes outbreaks of *acne vulgaris*, otherwise known as zits.

You sit under a blue light for fifteen minutes twice a week for eight weeks. By the end of treatment, your pores are bacteria-free, and no longer erupt into pimples. Monthly maintenance treatments will keep your skin clear. At forty dollars per session (you can buy more cost-effective packages), these facials won't break the bank. There's no downtime, no pain, and no risk.

If you have teenage daughters, I'd definitely recommend it for them, instead of painful extraction facials.

**Makeup palette.** "Makeup changes with the color of your clothes," Adele said. "If you're wearing a blue sweater, you can add just a hint of blue to the eyes, with liner or shadow. I do it because it matches my legs. If you're not sure what you're wearing, or you think you might change mid-day, stick with neutrals. On the face, use tans and taupes. On eyes, beiges and black. Put peach on the cheeks and go with rosy lips. This palette goes with anything."

**Lips.** "When you put on lip liner, keep your mouth in a natural closed position to see the shape you're making," said Adele. "So many women do it with their mouths open, with stretched-out lips. It's like drawing on a balloon, and then deflating it." Color-wise, for liner, choose a neutral to define the shape and a light rose color for inside. When your lips start to bleed color through the cracks, it's time to switch from red gloss to blendable neutral liners and lipsticks. You've got to tone it down as you get older. A slash of red was great in your twenties. But in your fifties, you don't want that Granny Goth look.

**Nose.** The nose can and should be contoured with makeup. First, Adele gives a good powdering and then uses a blend of brown and tan at the base and a soft, neutral, tan flesh tone on the sides and bridge, blended with her fingertip. This keeps the nose from shining, looking too pointy or wide.

**Chin.** Again, in that potentially shiny part, powder first with a soft, tan blend. Along the jaw, Adele uses a slightly darker shade to take away light reflection, making the line look sharper. She'll blend it down under the jaw, too. The whole area back to the base of the jaw gets shaded, taking away any hint of loose skin there.

**Cheeks.** The trick is to contour with a darker neutral just behind the molars. Add a blush on the apple of the cheek. Then, using light brushstrokes, sweep the color, almost invisibly, on the forehead, nose, and chin for a healthy glow. "I use high-quality brushes," said Adele. "Spending money on quality tools is as good an investment in makeup, as with anything else. You'll get better results, and the brushes last longer." A concert violinist uses a Stradivarius for a reason. Adele uses Trish McEvoy.

**Eyes.** Light shimmer is great for just under the eyebrow and in the inside corner of the eyes. Adele always uses neutral shadow on me, unless it's a red-carpet event and I'm wearing color.

Re: lashes, I've worn false lashes every day since 1969. I buy them in bulk, a hundred at a time. They really open the eye up. If you don't use fake ones, invest in good waterproof mascara. Or try the new formula that supposedly makes your lashes grow longer and thicker. It's called Marini Lash, made by Jan Marini. It's got a magic peptide that stimulates growth. I use it—I apply every night for a month—and I do see improvement. It's worth Googling.

Eyeliner should go along the upper lashline, and then it should sweep up. All makeup should be moving upward. I learned this on "The Ed Sullivan Show" a million years ago. It raises everything and creates the optical illusion of lift.

## Adele's Five-Minute Face

"A good time-saver is to use products that multitask, like a moisturizing foundation or a powder-based foundation," said Adele. "Next, fill in the eyebrows with a liner pencil. Put on some lipstick, mascara (or your false lashes), and a stroke of blush. Apply shadow if there's still time. If not, bring it with you and stroke it on at red lights or whenever you get a second in the course of the day. To start, though, as long as your eyes are defined with mascara and you've got color on your cheeks and lips, you'll have enough polish for the day."

Anyone can do it. It makes a huge psychological difference, like starting the day on the right foot. People will perceive you differently when you look put together. If you take the time to care for yourself, they owe you their respect.

Not wearing makeup is willfully taking yourself out of the game.

**Permanent Makeup.** The process of tattooing on eyeliner, eyebrows, or lip definition is called micropigmentation. It's just like regular tattooing—injecting colored ink into the dermal layer of skin with a needle—but on a small scale.

I have a lot of friends who've tried it. One had her lipline tattooed. The problem is that, over time, the tattoos become less defined. After a few years, they fade. On the eyes, this can be good, like a soft smudged liner. On the lips, though, you don't want a fuzzy line that looks like your hand was shaking when you put on your lipstick.

**Hair.** I do have thinning hair, but don't have the time for hair-transplant recovery. What I do instead is darken my scalp with makeup, so it doesn't shine through like a train coming out of a tunnel. A friend of mine had her scalp tattooed brown. The color faded over time, but that made it look even better, more natural. I wear mini extensions. It's a tiny ponytail of hair on a clip. I attached the clip to my other hair, and my mane looks filled out and thick.

Some do shake loose though. I'm constantly finding little hair clumps on the carpet. When guests come over, I just tell them the dog is shedding. So far, they haven't noticed I don't have a blond dog.

**Body.** Not to drum too loudly on this point, but women have to put in their time exercising. I hate it. I spend the first ten minutes of my workout trying to talk my trainer out of it. But, at the end of it, I'm glad I did it, not only for my figure but also for my health. Exercise helps prevent osteoporosis. It's good for the heart. It keeps you limber. I have several friends who are my age and can't walk up a flight of stairs. The ones who exercise are fine.

Besides my morning routine, I've made a habit of taking the stairs. If I drop something, I do a squat to pick it up. When I get off a plane, I walk through the terminal and avoid the moving platforms. And I push my own luggage cart, too. I secretly like it when the power goes out in my building and I have to walk up the eight flights of stairs to my apartment. My mother never exercised in a formal way, but she was running up and down the stairs of our house all day long.

If you want to walk at eighty, you have to take the stairs at fifty, sixty, and seventy. It's that simple.

**Clothes.** When you dress, show what you've got while you still can. When you get too old, you can't. There are two ways to go: you can dress for other women, or you can dress for men.

If you're dressing for women, you want to look chic.

For men, try to look hot, which means short, low-cut, tight, no stockings.

Men don't appreciate chic. They want to see breasts, ass, legs, bright colors. If you wear pink, it reminds them of a vagina.*

**Sexy Is Taking Care of Yourself.** Women want to feel good about themselves. And feeling sexy will do it. Beauty is in the eye of the beholder, and *you* are the beholder. At my age, all the men are too dead to behold anything. So you've got to please yourself.

All the procedures I've described in this book are aimed at just that. Feeling good about yourself. Even though plastic surgery has a long history—even though I have a long history with plastic surgery—I feel like this is just the start. Things are getting less and less invasive.

*Or, if they're gay, Liberace.

By the time this book comes out, six months from the time it was written, I'm sure there will be loads of new technologies and advances.

By the time my daughter Melissa's generation is starting to have things done, I bet plastic surgery will be *totally* non-invasive, that you really can have a lunchtime procedure that'll give you amazing results.

Remember that futuristic movie *Logan's Run*, where no one was allowed to live after age thirty? In the real future, no one alive will *look* like they're over thirty. We've come a long way since Dr. Frankenstein–type experimentation. One day soon, I'm sure, everyone will have the looks they want, and won't we all be happier for it?

**A Final Touch.** I've always said, "If everyone around the world got a nose job and lost twenty pounds, there'd be no wars." If you look good, you *feel* good. And if you feel good, who wants to fight? So there's my hidden agenda. I wanted to write this book to end war in my lifetime.

However, while I continue to work on my Nobel Peace Prize, hopefully, as a start, all this information given with much research, thought, and love will encourage you to feel good about yourself and know that you really can be the confident, beautiful woman you dream of being.

Like me.

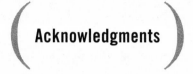

# Acknowledgments

I would not have been able to create this book (or my new face) without the help of a great many talented people . . . most of whom I am actually continuing to speak to.

Even though the idea to write a book about beauty through plastic surgery was right under my nose, it took mastermind, book packager, self-help author, and acclaimed film producer Larry Thompson to bring it to my attention. Before he finished pitching me the idea for this book (his wife, Kelly, actually had suggested the title), I said, "Yes! I'm absolutely passionate about this subject, and I think I know a thing or two or three about it, having been the poster child for plastic surgery since the invention of knives."

I am grateful to Larry not only for his ideas and creative talents, but also for his passion and confidence in me and all of my endeavors. Unlike all of the other stupid men in the world, he's drop-dead smart and a real visionary.

After our successful pre-op consultation, Larry and his most efficient head of development, Robert G. Endara II, discovered through literary agent Nancy Yost the brilliant researching skills and prolific writing talents of my co-writer, bestselling novelist, and new friend, Valerie Frankel.

In addition to researching and writing books (her newest is a memoir, *Thin Is the New Happy*), Val is also a sought-after magazine journalist. From 1990 to 2000, she was an articles editor at *Mademoiselle,* and during her tenure, she wrote monthly advice columns on sex, men, dating, etiquette, and female friendship. As a freelance writer, Val has been a fixture at *Parenting* and *Self,* as well as a contributor to nearly every major woman's magazine in the United States.

Thank you so, so much, Valerie.

Next, the literary agency Dupree Miller & Associates joined our efforts. They deserve many thanks. Jan Miller, a star maker and superstar herself, with her ever-vigilant and enthusiastic co-worker, Nena Madonia, went immediately to Simon & Schuster and inquired, "Would you like to offer entertaining and helpful information to all the women in the world?"

And then our vision became real.

With much enthusiasm, I want to thank everyone at Pocket Books and Simon & Schuster who rolled out the hospitality gurney for me. First, my deep appreciation goes to my glorious and talented editor, Mitchell Ivers, who embraced our proposal, smiled, and has escorted us every step of the way down the publishing red carpet. Also at Pocket Books and Simon & Schuster, big kisses and no small thanks to executive director Anthony Ziccardi and publisher Louise Burke, who also said "yes."

During the writing of this book, in addition to all the information I have gathered firsthand over the years from all the doctors I have interviewed or even used, we enlisted top plastic surgeons from across the country to serve on the book's advisory panel to guarantee 100 percent accuracy.

Robert Singer, M.D., F.A.C.S., past president of the American Society of Aesthetic Plastic Surgery, past chairman of the board for the American Society of Plastic Surgeons, current president of the American Association for Accreditation of Ambulatory Surgery Facilities Educational Foundation, has run a clinic in San Diego for thirty years. He's the industry spokesperson on public awareness and safety in his field. I met him doing a panel about plastic surgery on "Larry King Live," and he impressed me with his commitment and passion. The message he wants out there: plastic surgery *is* all that it's cracked up to be, as long you do the necessary homework about doctors, facilities, and procedures. Patients must make it their personal responsibility to be informed. I *completely* agree, and I want to thank him for giving his time and expertise in helping me in this book to go a long way toward that end.

Steven Hoefflin, M.D., F.I.C.S., F.A.C.S., the man who inspired the movie *Doc Hollywood*, has been my own surgeon for many years. He's worked on dozens of A-list stars, as well as tens of thousands of others at his Santa Monica–based Hoefflin Center for Plastic Surgery. Steve is the professional's professional, an author, a maverick, and an expert on the latest, greatest plastic surgery advances, tools, technology, and techniques.

Anthony Youn, M.D., a Rochester Hills, Michigan–based plastic surgeon who specializes in nose jobs, facial fillers, and eye lifts worked tirelessly with us on evenings and weekends.

Scott J. Zevon, M.D., is a Manhattan-based plastic surgeon who specializes in cosmetic plastic surgery of the face, breasts, and body. He loves his work and described six hours of surgery as "relaxing."

Lisa B. Cassileth, M.D., F.A.C.S., a Beverly Hills–based surgeon, specializes in breast surgery, body sculpting, and facial rejuvenation. Thanks to her, I can hold my arms high with pride when I give my grandson a high-five.

Shilesh Iyer, M.D., a Manhattan-based dermatologist who specializes in skin resurfacing, laser surgery, liposuction, Botox therapy, soft-tissue augmentation, and skin cancer surgery, works endlessly at making sure that all of the correct information is given to patients.

David Louis Matlock, M.D., M.B.A., F.A.C.O.G., based in Los Angeles, is the pioneer of the trademarked procedures Laser Vaginal Rejuvenation® and the G-Shot®. He is the founder and medical director of the Laser Vaginal Rejuvenation Institute of America.

And finally, Jerome Spivack, M.D., a plastic surgeon based in Westfield, New Jersey, who generously gave his time and expertise. Thanks, Jerry!

That's quite a team. . . . Thank you all for your advice and dedicated work.

I sincerely want to say thanks to my personal manager and cheerleader, Billy Sammeth, my agent, Joel Dean, my entertainment attorney, Kenneth Browning, my business manager, Michael Karlin, my indefatigable personal assistant, Jocelyn Pickett, and my longtime publicist, Judy Katz. With that payroll, you know why I work my ass off.

I also want to thank every woman who has ever stopped me and asked me about plastic surgery. All of you confirmed for me the need to research and get out all the truthful and comprehensive information about beauty procedures available today.

And lastly, a special thank-you to my one and only darling daughter, Melissa, and her adorable son, Cooper, for allowing me to embark on yet another creative effort that robs us of our precious time together. To Melissa, who calls me by the most beautiful name in the world, "Mom," and to my grandson, Cooper, who refers to me after each of my beauty enhancements as "Nana New Face," I want to say, thank you for everything and I love you very much. You both really do make me feel blessed and beautiful.